Preventing Dementia, Naturally:

Assuring the healthy child, adult, and senior throughout the generations

By Dr. Danielle West-Stellick, ND
Doctor of Naturopathy

Lariat Publishing

ISBN: 978-1-887219-41-9
Published in the United States of America

Table of Contents

Introduction

When I told a dear friend of mine that I was working on this book, she asked more about what it was about. And when I told her, she was amazing: "You mean you can prevent dementia?" My response of course was "Yes, and you can break the generational curse dementia carries with it, and THAT IS what the book is all about!" Needless to say, she was astounded!

Two months ago I published *Fear of Forgetting* and *My Life, My Memories,* two interactive books for the patient in the early stage of one of the dementias or Alzheimer's disease. Fear of Forgetting contained a brief discussion on the health-related risk factors associated with the development of dementia, such as obesity, diabetes, high blood pressure, and a life of heavy metal exposure. Chapter Three explores these risk factors, and more, in greater depth. If you know the risk factors, and can mitigate your risk, then the potential for that problem developing significantly lessens. That is a basic premise no matter what a risk is attached to.

In the case of risks of developing dementia are concerned, knowing the risks and mitigating them is critical.

Not counting all other forms of dementia, Alzheimer's disease alone currently affects 5.5 million people in the US, with an anticipated rise to 16 million by the year 2050. If more people focused on prevention, whether as an adult, or by instilling healthy habits in children that are maintained into adulthood, even now with 33 years to go until 2050, I believe that total number of individuals diagnosed with Alzheimer's disease in the US would be dramatically less than 16 million people! Not only that, but as I was literally completing my final edits on this book, an article came out in the New England Journal of Medicine - Journal Watch Neurology that stated the death rate due to Alzheimer's disease alone increased by more than 50% in just 15 years, from1999 to 2015. That's in increase in less than a generation's time!

Think about the numbers for a minute and the impact of that dramatic growth projected over the next 33 years; the growth basically describes dementia affecting the next generation. Sadly, as this book will bring out in Chapter Four, the critical risk factors associated with the development of dementia are not just issues one deals with in their adult years; they are rapidly increasing in numbers as affecting children too. In fact, type 2 diabetes is affecting children in epidemic proportions.

Therefore, rather than focusing on prevention of dementia being strictly something to pay attention to as an adult, which I believe is pivotal in our day and age, I strongly believed a discussion of how effective healthcare starting in childhood is the ultimate preventative mechanism necessary to stop the growth pattern of diseases like Alzheimer's.

Please take my words to heart. I strongly believe that together we can help restore you to a healthier adult and prevent the onset of dementia or Alzheimer's disease in our current generation, and in you. But I also believe that by paying attention to what happens to our children, and to our children's children, and looking at some of the risk patterns that are established from childhood on which foster the risks associated with the onset of dementia in old age, risks can be mitigated and fewer of today's children will run the risk of becoming a statistic.

Together, let's focus on alleviating the risk factors, such as obesity, high blood pressure, high cholesterol, cardiovascular disease, atherosclerosis, diabetes, and heavy metal or chemical toxicity. And together, let's break the link of generational suffering as the risk of dementia is present from parent to child.

Chapter One: The brain

The human brain is an amazing, incredibly complex, part of our body. In order to understand how issues with risk factors affect the brain and lead to dementia, or specifically Alzheimer's disease, this chapter is going to offer a brief anatomical profile of the human brain. This and the next chapter, which goes into the finer aspects of the neurology of the brain, and how this is affected in dementia, and specifically Alzheimer's disease will the aerial on risk factors make more sense than if I just launched right in with that as our first chapter. So please bear with me. I promise to make this as painless as possible for you!

In each of the three dementia disorders, the brain is the area affected. The figure below is a very basic diagram of one side of your brain. Remember, there are two sides, the right and the left, so some of the lobes, or sections of the brain I'll discuss also have right and left sections.

Figure 1[1]

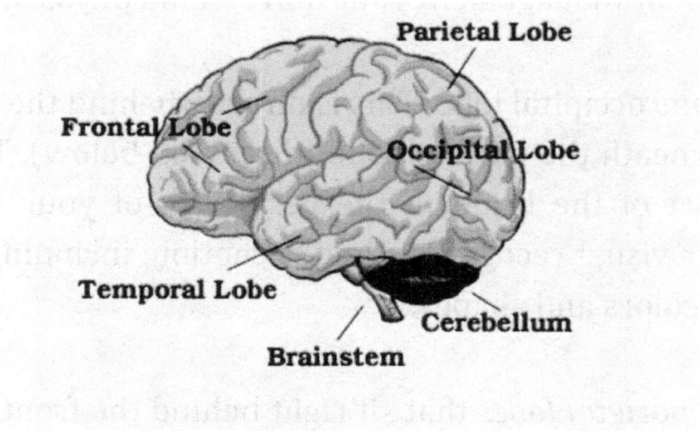

[1] Johnson, G. (2014). Understanding the Principle Lobes of the Brain. Brain Injury Help. http://braininjuryhelp.com/principal-lobes-of-the-brain/

There is only one brainstem. The *brainstem* connects the brain to the spinal cord, essentially providing the neural pathway between the brain and the body. Functionally, the brainstem provides us with the mechanisms for basic survival, for example, breathing, digestion, blood pressure, heart rate, and wakefulness.

There is only one cerebellum. This section lies at the very bottom of the brain, just behind the brain stem. The *cerebellum* is the area of the brain responsible for coordination, including both muscle coordination and balance. Functionality associated with the cerebellum includes walking, talking, eating, and many self-care tasks.

There is only *one* frontal lobe. As the name implies, it is in the front of the brain. The *frontal lobe*, has two sections. The front is often referred to as the *prefrontal cortex* (but don't be confused, just think front part of the frontal lobe), and is where functioning related to your personality resides, as well as those neurological activities responsible for higher cognitive thinking. The *back* section of the frontal lobe is where premotor and motor areas reside, and controls your ability to change position or management your movements physically.

There is only *one* occipital lobe. This is directly behind the frontal lobe, and just underneath the parietal lobe (discussed below). The *occipital lobe* is the part of the brain in the very back of your skull that is responsible for visual recognition and reception, including being able to distinguish colors and shapes.

There are two *parietal lobes* that sit right behind the frontal lobe, with one on each side of the brain. Each of the two parietal lobes have different functions. The *right parietal lobe* is responsible for making sense of visuo-spatial input, for example, finding your way around familiar places, or even new places. The left parietal lobe is like the language center of your brain, helping you understand the written or spoken word. Both parietal lobes contain primary sensory areas that help us interpret basic sensations such as pressure, or touch. Still within each parietal lobe, but tucked behind this basic sensory section is another area that helps control finer sensory awareness, for example, assessment of size, shape, weight, and interpretation of texture.

There are also two *temporal lobes*, one on each side of the brain. The temporal lobes are also responsible for sensory activity, primarily related to scent and sound, and both are involved in short-term memory. The *right temporal lobe* is involved in visual memory, for example face or picture recognition. The *left temporal lobe* is involved in verbal memory, for example names, verbal labels, and other words.

One more critical part of the brain is the *hippocampus*, as shown in Figure 2 below. The hippocampus is responsible for the formation of new memories and has also been reported by some to be a gateway of sorts into the formation of more permanent memories. As you might suspect, the hippocampus is one of the first areas of the brain that will evidence damage from dementia or Alzheimer's disease.

Now that we understand a little about the brain structure and the very basic functions of each area, what are dementia, Alzheimer's disease, and Mild Cognitive Impairment? And, what actually happens when these occur?

Figure 2[2]

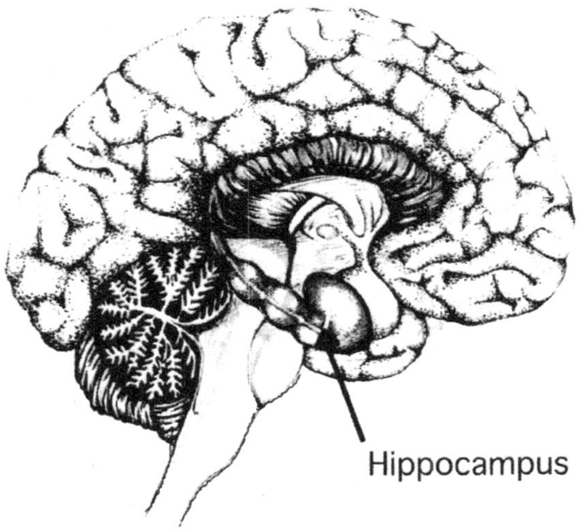

[2] Myers, A. (2000). In Catherine Myers' Memory Loss and the Brain. Retrieved from http://www.memorylossonline.com/glossary/hippocampus.html

Chapter Two: Dementia, Alzheimer's disease, and Mild Cognitive Impairment

Each of these three disorders: dementia, Alzheimer's disease, and Mild Cognitive Impairment share commonalities and present with differences. This chapter will focus strictly on the facts. Sadly, as statistics bear out, Alzheimer's disease and varied dementias affect so many older individuals today, the inclination is to immediately panic and freeze as soon as we hear the phrase; it's almost as if a death sentence has been pronounced upon the patient. In many ways, the diagnosis of Alzheimer's disease or dementia of any type creates an even greater fear to the patient and their family members than would a diagnosis of cancer.

Many have heard they either have one of these disorders, are caring for someone with one of these disorders, or have heard the phrases but really don't fully understand what the diagnosis involves and why the disorder progresses as it does. In other words, they don't truly know what is really happening to the person's body.

What is dementia?

The thing about dementia is that it is a generalized diagnosis, it is a collective term rather than a specific disease. Therefore, this brief section will detail the various major types of dementia that are associated with the symptoms commonly seen in patients one associates with Alzheimer's, such as the gradual loss of memory and cognitive skills. Of those that we'll discuss here, Alzheimer's disease accounts for 60 to 80 percent of cases. Vascular dementia is the second most common dementia type. Although not a disease, but a classification, at least two of the following list of core mental functions must be significantly impaired before a diagnosis of dementia to be made:

- Memory loss – usually short-term memory, but can progress to long-term memory as well;
- Problems with communication and language, most evident first in speech;
- Inability to focus and pay attention;

- Faulty reasoning and judgment, for example forgetting that hot means hot;
- Disruptions in visual perception, including hallucinations.

As I stated above, there are a number of types of dementia, but rather than confuse you with dementia that is primarily related to other disease challenges, let's talk about the four primary types that you are most likely to hear discussed when concerned about the potential for Alzheimer's disease, memory loss, and aging.

Alzheimer's disease

Alzheimer's disease: the phrase that instantly strikes fear in anyone 55 and above. In fact, most cases of dementia are simply referred to as Alzheimer's disease by people who don't realizes there is a difference in the underlying physiological issue because memory is affected in each type of dementia. Even many adult residential settings refer to their extended care wing as the "Alzheimer's Wing." This could be due to the sad reality that Alzheimer's disease is the most common type of dementia affecting between 60 – 80% of those with any form of dementia. In fact, as of this writing, Alzheimer's is affecting some 5 million individuals aged 65 or older. That translates into one out of every nine individuals aged 65 or older being a victim of Alzheimer's disease; which is tragic. Additionally, Alzheimer's can strike those younger than 65 years of age through the early onset of the disorder (still different than Mild Cognitive Impairment), and popularized in the movie *Still Alice* with Julianne More. In fact, statistical for this year tell us that early onset Alzheimer's disease currently affects 200,000 younger patients.

The most common symptoms associate with Alzheimer's disease is that the patient displays difficulty remembering anything recent (short-term), including conversations, names or events. Other symptoms that might also present with short term memory problems including apathy and depression. As the disorder progresses through the four general stages, symptoms that you might be more familiar with when thinking of the patient with Alzheimer's (or for that matter all dementias in their later stages) include impaired communication, poor judgment, disorientation, confusion, behavior changes and difficulty speaking, swallowing and walking.

Many of you may have heard the term plaque, usually thinking of the arteries in your heart. The classic physiological problems that differentiate the diagnosis of Alzheimer's disease from the physiological changes seen in other dementias is the deposit of plaque (beta-amyloid) as well as what are referred to as tangles, which are simply twisted strands of a specific protein (tau). Additionally, Alzheimer's disease presents with very clear damage to nerve cells and actual cell death in the brain.

From the nerve cell diagram below you can see there are four distinct parts of the cell: the cell body (soma), the dendrites, the axon, and the axon terminals (technically part of the axon). Nerve impulses occur in the synapse, which is the place where nerve cells meet each other, as the axon terminals fire towards the dendrites of the adjacent nerve cell. As shown in Figure 4 below, nerve cells become damaged, often at the dendrites, and thus make communication between nerve cells difficult at best. Figure 4 shows what it looks like amidst nerve cells trying to communicate with damaged dendrites, and with tangles and plaque present.

If that seems a little confusing, think of it this way. Nerve cells can be visualized as an elliptical cell, with a tail at one end that is called the axon which lead to the axon terminals that fire nerve impulses to the next nerve cell. The central part of the nerve cell itself has what look like tentacles coming off of it; these are called dendrites. These receive the impulses sent to the cell from the axon terminals of another nerve cell when firing. When nerve cells become damaged, as is the case as dementia or Alzheimer's disease progress, dendrites are damaged, making communication between nerve cells difficult – it simply can't receive the communication from the firing cell. Additionally, as the diseases progress and nerve cells are damaged, tangles and plaque form on the axonal terminals, making firing difficult or impossible.

As the disease and damage progress, it becomes harder and harder and harder for nerve cells to communicate, and as a result, nerve cells die off. If you look at a slide of brain tissue under a microscope, there are fewer nerve cells in the same tissue section when Alzheimer's disease is present. Therefore, in addition to damaged dendrites, because of the dead nerve cells (which continue to die in increasing numbers as the disease progresses), those that remain are farther apart.

Figure 3[3]

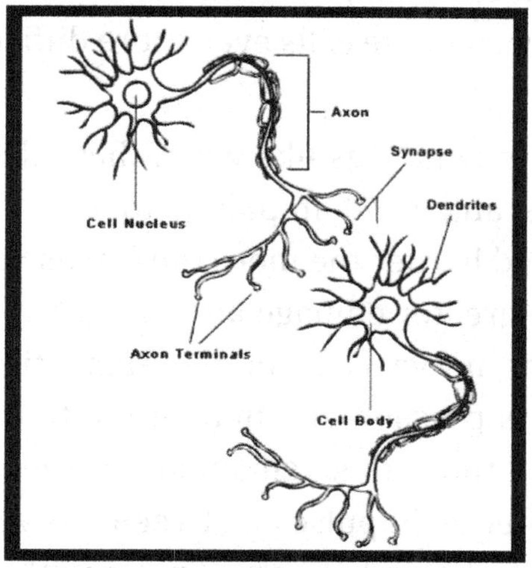

Figure 4[4]

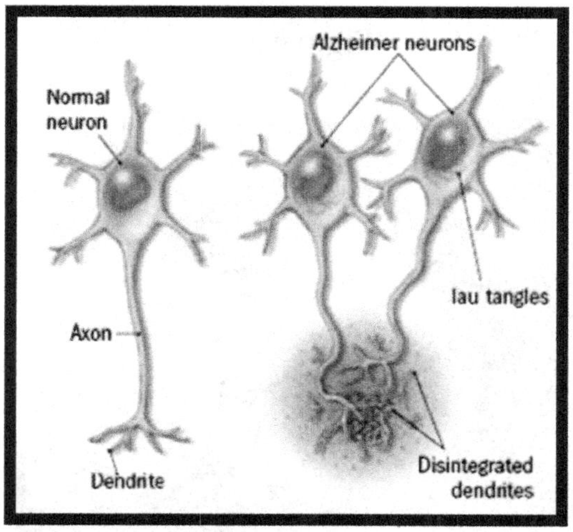

[3] Koch, S. (n.d.). My Brain Notes.com. Retrieved from http://mybrainnotes.com/brain-cortex-neurons.html
[4] Murphy, M. (n.d.). RadioKinesis. Retrieved from http://kinesiologydatabase.com/page/view/how-the-brain-works

The result of all of these changes is that it makes communication of nerve impulses between nerve cells even more difficult.

Figure 5 below shows what it is like when these damaged nerve cells try to communicate and send impulses to each other. It becomes harder and harder and harder the more the disease progresses and the nerve cells evidence greater damage and ultimately death. As you can see, there are fewer nerve cells in the same tissue section when Alzheimer's disease is present, and in addition to damaged dendrites, many simply die, and those that remain are farther apart. This makes communication of nerve impulses between nerve cells even more difficult; like the old fashioned electrical poles with wires that you still may see in some areas. The wires had to connect with each other to complete the circuit. If there is nothing to connect with, the signal does not go through.

Figure 5[5]

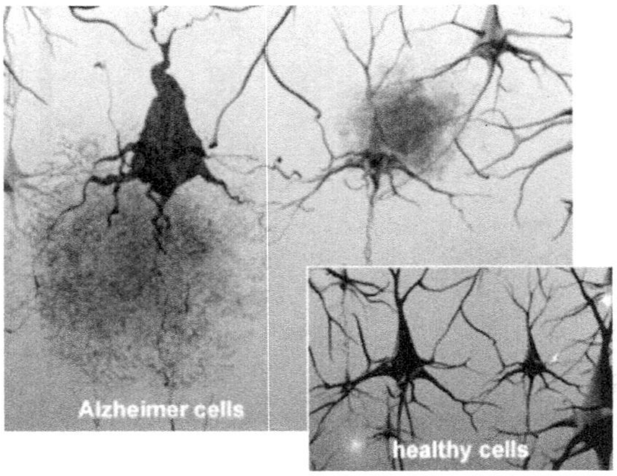

[5] Alzheimer's Association. (2011). Retrieved from https://www.alz.org/braintour/plaques_tangles.asp

Sadly, the combination of these neurological events leads to the brain actually shrinking and, for lack of a better word, eroding. You can see the differences of Alzheimer's both in size when comparing the healthy brain to one with severe Alzheimer's disease, as well as the areas affected as the disease progresses showing the degradation in the brain itself by comparing the limited areas affected and minimal shrinkage in the early stage compared to the multiple lobes affected and significant shrinkage by the time the patient is in the later, severe/late stage of Alzheimer's disease. As the disease progresses, healthy brain tissue reduces in size and the quality of remaining brain tissue is significantly compromised, with specific damage to lobes evident in the stage-based discussion that follows.

Stages of Alzheimer's

It is pretty well established that the symptoms of Alzheimer's disease worsen over time, although the rate at which the disease progresses varies, as does longevity following diagnosis. Longevity is based on a number factors thus there is a wide range with some living as little as four years and others living as long as 20 years. Therefore, as I detail the major stages of Alzheimer's disease below, I will also give average lengths that the stage lasts. Understand just as longevity depends on the individual, so does the rate of progression from one stage to the next.

As you might imagine, there are microscopic and biochemical changes deep inside the brain that affect the nerve cells themselves due to Alzheimer's disease itself which start the cascade, in a pre-clinical stage which can last for many years. I've chosen not to discuss that stage here in detail as symptoms can mirror those of other chronic diseases, depression, or even fatigue. However, it is important to know that the symptoms are virtually impossible to detect without the use of specialized and costly diagnostic imaging examinations, and most individuals at this pre-clinical stage stage would still pass the classic dementia or Alzheimer's disease memory tests.

The number of stages one passes through as the disease progresses are varied in number based on who you are talking to from three to seven. Typically, when people talk about more stages, they are breaking down the major ones we're going to discuss into subsets. For our purposes here, we'll just talk about the four major stages: early, moderate, moderate to severe, and severe. Given we've just talked about the structure of the brain, Figure 6 below highlights the differences and damage to the brain as each stage of Alzheimer's, for example, progresses.

Figure 6[6]

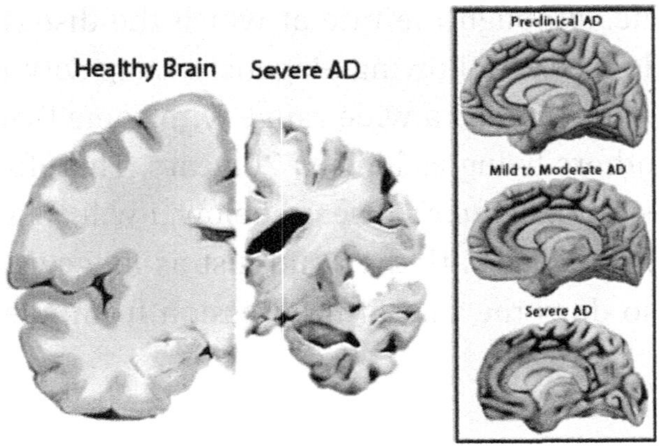

---

[6] Shiel, W. (2016). Dementia, Alzheimer's and Aging Brains. Retrieved from http://www.onhealth.com/content/1/dementia_memory_brain_disorder

The Mild/Early Stage of Alzheimer's

Unlike the preclinical stage, when an individual actually enters the initial mild or early stage of Alzheimer's disease, a conclusive diagnosis can generally be made. One of the most common symptoms displayed is the inability to handle complex activities typically associated with daily life events, such as balancing their checkbook, or going to the grocery store. Short-term memory is also affected and will be evident to others in this stage as well. For example, it is not uncommon for patients to claim no memory of recent activities or conversations, remember the names of new people after an initial introduction, even forgetting something they just read.

Those interacting with the patient might also notice mood changes. For example, the person might seem withdrawn. They may be less emotionally present or reactive. And pivotal here for caretakers and patients is the notion that although a person may be aware of their new deficits, a very strong feature usually seen is denial. Remember, this is a frightening diagnosis affecting so many that even thinking about the future for some creates a sense of immediate fear and doom. These feelings may also cause the patient to withdraw from family events or other regular activities because they don't want others to notice the very changes that they themselves fear. To have others see the changes makes it all the more real and painful. There may also be a perceived social stigma attached to the dementia or Alzheimer's disease diagnosis also leading to social withdrawal and isolation.

All is not lost however. During the mild or early stage, patients can generally remember important things, such as the name of the president, current events, their address, and similar concepts and facts. And despite the overt cognitive challenges affecting the patient, most individuals can still maintain their own independence, drive safely, and care for themselves, but others often transition into a residential community setting.

The early/mild stage generally lasts an average of two years. Therefore, it strongly behooves the patient to use that time, once a diagnosis is made, to use that time to the fullest and make all appropriate plans for the future for themselves and family members.

The Moderate Stage of Alzheimer's

The next stage, when one is considered to have Moderate Alzheimer's, can last for many years with the patient requiring increasing levels of care. Typically, patients in this stage live in a full-time residential setting or are dependent upon a full-time caregiver such as a child or spouse. Caregivers make certain the patient is eating properly and taking their medication as prescribed, that they are properly dressed, and that personal hygiene is maintained. Without constant care in the moderate stage, many patients might wear the same clothes for days or weeks at a time if left to their own devices.

Cognitively, patients in the moderate stage at this stage frequently cannot remember many of the things they still could in the mild/early stage, such as their address or who the president is, and memories associated with various part of their personal life begins to become more selective in nature. Additionally, rather than only short-term memory being affected, by the time the patient enters the moderate stage of Alzheimer's disease, long-term, or remote memory, becomes affected as well.

Other cognitive changes also demonstrate the continued neural erosion, as normal calculations frequently cannot be performed, for example, requesting the patient count backwards from 20 by 2s presents difficulty. Therefore, if the individual is still living independently, and not in a residential center, it is common for caregivers monitor that payment are paid. Emotional changes are also very common, with patients in the moderate stage of Alzheimer's disease to demonstrate increased level of suspicion, confusion, fear, anger, and behaving in generally uncharacteristic ways. The increased neurological damage that spread to more of the lobes in the brain underlie many of the increased emotional and cognitive problems evidenced by the patient. Sadly, often patients are unable to properly express their feelings or thoughts by the time they are in the moderate stage or about to transition into the moderate/severe stage.

Other symptoms that will become evident when the patient has transitioned from the mild/early stage of Alzheimer's disease into the moderate stage include: growing incontinence; reversing the normal sleep pattern, for example sleeping during the day and wandering at night; easily becoming lost and disoriented; and the onset of repetitive behaviors, for example shredding tissues or wringing their hands.

The Moderate to Severe Stage of Alzheimer's

In the Moderate to Severe stage, the patient is typically neurologically compromised to the point where they can no longer perform basic daily tasks. As I discuss this major stage, know that there are subtle shifts within this third major stage until the patient is officially classified as in the Severe stage.

For example, at early of the Moderate to Severe stage, patients may have difficulty getting dressed and not know what do to with their clothing. They may even put on multiple layers of the incorrect clothing on, such as pajamas on over their day clothes. This is frequently one of the signs most noted in the official transition from the moderate to the moderate to severe stage. Personal hygiene and the general mechanics of toileting may cause problems. For example, patients are likely to forget to flush the toilet and may not dispose of toilet tissue properly. As the stage progresses, patients will become increasingly incontinent, with urinary incontinence affecting the patient prior to fecal incontinence. (This should not be confused with incontinence that may be associated with aging due to weak pelvic floor muscles). As patients enter the moderate to severe stage and the disease progresses from a neurological perspective affecting more of the lobes in the brain, sensory perceptions relative to temperature are affected, often creating problems for bathing as the patient cannot properly adjust the water temperature.

Cognitively, as the decline in memory continues in the moderate to severe stage, the patient displays little awareness of their life events, may confuse family members for one another, such as a mother for a wife or even those who are already deceased, and ultimately speech becomes extremely minimal or may cease completely. In addition to memory issues, simple cognitive functions are severely compromised as well. For example, even well educated patients cannot count backwards from 10.

Emotionally, patients in the moderate to severe stage present with some of the most disturbing aspects of Alzheimer's disease, particularly for caretakers. Although much is the result of physiological loss in the brain itself, a lot of behavioral issues in the patient are due to displaced levels of energy, much as they would be in a young child. For example, since the patient can no longer participate in activities they used to, they now displace that energy and are likely to fidget or pace as if those actions are the most important for the patient to do at that moment, whether appropriate or not. Although verbal communication is limited, and often stuttering is seen, outbursts are also frequently witnessed as patients adopt violent or threatening behaviors to cope with their fears. Personally, I believe this is more than a coping mechanism, I believe it is the patients way of trying to communicate in the only manner they can that something is wrong. For example, my mother used to scratch and bite my brother constantly in outbursts of anger. I believe she was trying to tell him something in the only way she could, even though to my brother, it was viewed as aggressive and violent behavior that he didn't understand. Typically, the moderate stage as a whole lasts just shy of 2.5 years before the patient enters the severe/late stage of Alzheimer's disease.

The Severe/Late Stage of Alzheimer's

In the final stage of this disease, individuals lose the ability to respond to their environment, to carry on a conversation and, eventually, to control their movement. They may still say words or phrases on random occasions, but communicating pain becomes difficult and eventually ceases completely. As memory and cognitive skills continue to worsen, further personality changes may take place and individuals need extensive help with daily activities. Like all the stages of the disease, this last stage is progressive, and has its own clear demarcations of the final disease path.

Initially verbal communication may be limited to approximately a half dozen intelligible words or fewer, and these are only spoken when intensive contact is initiated with the patient. As the patient progresses through this stage, speech becomes more limited to perhaps only one remaining word, before the capacity for speech is completely lost. By the time the capacity for verbal communication is lost, the patient rapidly loses the ability to walk without assistance, and ultimately to walk at all. Patients may have difficult remaining upright when seated if in a chair without arm rests or unless they have a type of chest strap for use when seated in a chair. Patients may also display difficulty holding their head upright. Again, I refer you to the figures earlier in this section and the discussion on the various lobes in the brain so that you can see why the patient is losing these various capacities.

As a result of the widespread brain damage, the physical changes can be startling to those who perceive of Alzheimer's disease as strictly one affecting the brain. On the one hand, that is correct; it does affect the brain. However, the brain is the center of regulating all bodily activity. Therefore, with increasing brain damage, functionality is lost in addition to memory or cognition. For example, in the later phases of this final stage, range of motion is exchanged with joint rigidity and resistance. This is often a sign that further irreversible physical deformity known as contractures which prevent any range of motion without inflicting severe pain upon movement are soon to follow. Contractures in major joints affected upwards of 40% of Alzheimer's patients in the severe/late stage of their disease, however if the patient is already immobile, contractures are known to afflict upwards of 95% of late stage Alzheimer's disease.

In the end, the most common cause of death in the Alzheimer's patient is pneumonia, often from aspiration, as their bodily functions literally do not have the neurological component to function. However, statistically, those with Alzheimer's are evidenced in academic literature as being more vulnerable to the effects of other life-threatening diseases, including heart attack, stroke, and cancer.

Vascular dementia

Only accounting for 10% of the cases, vascular dementia is significantly less common than Alzheimer's disease. Other names for vascular dementia that you might have heard or that your doctor might use are post-stroke or multi-infarct dementia. Multi-infarct refers to damage resulting from multiple strokes, or interruptions to the blood flow of the brain. Whereas Alzheimer's disease is progressive in a more gradual manner, vascular dementia from a vascular dementia is also progressive, but can be viewed as a stairway, with each step down a very very very long flight of stairs, or multiple flights of stairs, each being damage from a stroke in a progression of strokes. Many strokes evidenced in vascular dementia are imperceptible, however, they usually occur without the typical aphasia, paralysis, or facial distortion one commonly associates with stroke victims.

Typical symptoms associated with vascular dementia include impaired judgment and planning before evidencing a decline in memory. For example, the ability to organize or plan activities might present a problem and become a source of frequent frustration. This can be contrasted with Alzheimer's disease where problems with memory are typically the first symptom.

Physiologically, the changes resulting from vascular dementia are a result of damage from blocked blood vessels during the stroke. Damage can also result from bleeding in the brain. The specific location where the stroke occurs, coupled with the size of the injury, and number of times the blood flow is blocked or bleeding into the brain occurs will impact the actual destructive nature of the brain injury. Based on the degree of stroke-related injury, this determines how the individual's thinking and physical functioning are affected.

Dementia with Lewy bodies

Another type of dementia is referred to as dementia with Lewy bodies. Lewy bodies are clusters of a specific type of protein (alpha-synuclein, which is found in abundance throughout the brain) that bind together when they should not. Although the individual with dementia with Lewy bodies will initially present with memory problems like Alzheimer's disease, other symptoms that will also likely present in the very early stages include insomnia or other sleep-related problems, visual hallucinations, and display some symptoms in common with Parkinson's disease, such as problems with balance when walking.

Mixed dementia

In mixed dementia, abnormalities are linked to more than one cause of dementia, that occur simultaneously in the brain. In fact, the biggest challenge of diagnosing dementia with Lewy bodies is that symptoms can appear the same as those with either vascular dementia or Alzheimer's disease. Symptoms can actually be from the physiological causes of dementia with Lewy bodies, AND vascular dementia AND Alzheimer's disease all contributing to the underlying dementia itself. In this case the diagnosis is referred to as mixed dementia. It is interesting to note that increased medical and academic research in this area demonstrates that most dementia patients are suffering from mixed dementia rather than a single type as previously thought.

Mild Cognitive Impairment

Affecting approximately 10 – 15% of individuals over the age of 65, many physicians refer to *Mild Cognitive Impairment* as symptomatic pre-dementia. I personally don't care for that term as it implies an automatic transition into a more serious progressive dementia of one type or another, which is not necessarily the case. The former does not necessitate the later. Although the medical research supports my opinion, this is frequently a cause of debate among neurologists.

Mild cognitive impairment, however, presents like pre-clinical or very very early stages of Alzheimer's disease. Mild cognitive impairment causes cognitive changes that are serious enough to be noticed by the individuals experiencing them or to other people, but the changes are not severe enough to interfere with daily life or independence.

Mild Cognitive Impairment is typically classified based on the skills affected, whether memory only referred to as *amnestic*, cognition only referred to as *non-amnestic*, or both. Typical amnestic challenges present when the patient starts to forget important information that he or she would previously have recalled easily, such as appointments, conversations or recent events. Non-amnestic symptoms typically include judgment impairments. For example, individuals may not make appropriate decisions, or they may have problems completing complex tasks.

One of the key ways Mild Cognitive Impairment presents itself is by cognitive (and/or memory specific) losses that are atypical than what might normally be associated with the patient's age or educational background. In the case of multiple assessments conducted by a psychiatrist or neurologist over a period of several months, the cognitive and/or memory challenges in patients with mild cognitive impairment will a show progressive decline. During this time, patients my may require additional time to complete tasks, function at a reduced level of efficiency, and simply make mistakes on things they normally wouldn't have in the past. However, the majority of functions associated with daily life, including not only self-care, but paying bills, grocery shopping, meal preparation, and so forth can still generally be performed without need of assistance. In fact, individuals can typically continue their normal work and social lives uninterrupted. On occasion, the individual may only require minimal assistance.

I believe at this point you should understand the significant of how complex the brain is, and how devastating the effects of dementia, and in particular Alzheimer's disease, is on the anatomy and physiology of the human brain. So let's examine the risk factors that lead the body on a cascade of health changes that bring about this devastation, and then we can look at how to naturally prevent the risks! This is a case of the best defense is a good offense!

Chapter Three: Risk factors

What is it that I really mean when I talk about risk factors? Technically, risk factors are those events associated with the onset or occurrence of something. In medical terms, that is interpreted as a risk factor associated with the onset or occurrence of a disorder or disease state.

Typically, risk factors are determined through statistical analysis that draws the correlation, or association, between one given situation and the onset or occurrence of another. For example, one of the greatest risk factors associated with the onset of Alzheimer's disease is advanced age. Well, we said in the last chapter the onset of Alzheimer's disease is highly correlated to those aged 65 or older, where one in nine individuals are diagnosed (roughly 11%) with the disease, whereas by age 85 that figure increases to one in three individuals (roughly 33.3%). Age is also considered a major risk factor for the onset of other dementias, particularly vascular dementia, due to the increase in coronary artery disorders as an individual age. However, the important thing to make note of here, and I urge you highlight this next phrase: *A risk factor does not in and of itself cause the occurrence of a correlated disease or disorder!*

Now, a little side note: Before I became a doctor, I was in operations and project management in the corporate environment. One of my favorite parts of the job was risk management. In risk management, an individual brainstorms and lists all the possible risks associated with a project or task and puts them in a spreadsheet or risk management program. Then they look at what the consequences of the risk are, usually associating a time and dollar amount to each possible consequence. At this point you have your risk assessment list.

But awareness of your list, your assessment alone, is only the beginning of the story. From there, there are mitigation strategies that need be developed, costs associated with mitigation strategies, and risks associated with those, etc. And then, you continue to monitor your risk assessment list on a daily, weekly, or monthly basis depending on the task or project length.

We can liken that to what we're about to do here. This chapter will present the risk assessment portion. In our next chapters we'll talk about mitigation strategies! And, as you'll see, just like in life, your health is the same. There are some things that you cannot change, and then there are others that you can. In our mitigation strategies, we'll focus on what you can change. But for this assessment presentation, you need to know and be aware of ALL the risk factors!

For our discussion, you should recognize that there are two kinds of risks: non-modifiable, and modifiable. Non-modifiable risks are those that the individual cannot change. They are a given, they are fixed. Modifiable risk factors associated with Alzheimer's disease are those that an individual can change through modifications in their diet, lifestyle, or through other means.

Risk factors associated with dementias

Ethnicity. Similar to the increased risk for Alzheimer's in individuals of Western origin, some ethnicities have an increased risk associated with specific cardiovascular diseases automatically putting them at risk for one of the dementias, particularly vascular dementia. This is the case for those of South Asian orientation, including those of India and Pakistan where there is a higher risk of diabetes, stroke, and heart disease than in many other cultures. Other ethnic groups are also at a higher risk of developing dementia, such as those of African or African-

Caribbean origin, risk due to their increased risk of diabetes and stroke.

Medical conditions. The majority of medical conditions that are linked to an increase in the risk factors associated with the onset of any one of the dementias include atherosclerosis, which is a thickening and hardening of arterial walls due to the build up of plaque, which ultimately limits blood flow by narrowing the available passageway for blood to flow throughout the body, including the brain.

Given the association between atherosclerosis and cholesterol, high LDL cholesterol levels are also considered a high risk factor for the onset of one of the dementias. The same is true for homocysteine, which is a protein that acts to repair damage to damaged arteries from plaque buildup. If there is plaque build up, the body will automatically evidence higher levels of homocysteine. As a result, homocysteine levels are considered a marker for risk factors associated with cardiovascular disease. Therefore, when normal cardiac risk blood panels are performed, doctors usually check for levels of homocysteine.

Smoking cessation is critical for the prevention of dementia. For example, cigarette smoking is associated with a higher risk of developing atherosclerosis and other types of vascular diseases, which in turn contribute to the increased risk of dementia. In particular, most of the time we only think about the risks of cigarette smoking in relation to respiratory issues; this is simply shortsighted. The truth is that cigarette smoking harms nearly every organ of the body, causes many diseases, and has significant circulatory and cardiopulmonary consequences. How does this relate to dementia? Smoking damages blood vessels and can make them thicken and grow narrower. Every time you smoke a cigarette, your heart beats faster and your blood pressure rises; creating a cycle ultimately reducing circulation, especially to your arms, legs, skin, and even the brain, and can form clots, this increasing the risk of stroke (a blood clot or burst blood vessel in or around the brain) and cardiovascular disease by two to four times the rate of non-smokers. Smoking is also associated with Smoking is a cause of type 2 diabetes mellitus and can make it harder to control, increasing the risk of developing type 2 diabetes at a rate 30–40% higher than nonsmokers. Remember these are all significant risk factors associated with the onset of dementia.

Obesity. Maintaining a healthy weight is equally important. Like cigarette smoking, being overweight or obese is a critical risk factor for the what I refer to as the triple crown of chronic diseases: high blood pressure, high cholesterol, and diabetes. If you are overweight, and you have one of these disorders, the risks are significantly higher that you will develop the others; it's just a matter of time. There was a time when weight charts were standardized to age and skeletal frame, such as small boned, medium, or large. Now, weight charts go by body mass indexes (BMI) calculated off your weight and height for the determination of whether you are obese or not. Underweight is classified as a height weight calculation <18.5; normal weight is a BMI in the range of 18.5–24.9; a person is classified as overweight if their BMI is between 25–29.9; and they are classified as obesity with a BMI of 30 or greater. For example, even a big boned man who is 5'11" weighing 212 pounds has a BMI of 29.6, which is very close to the cut off between overweight and obese. In other words, the person many not even look very large, certainly not what we might consider obese for the physiological risks to be present. If you want to check our own status, a very simple online calculator can be found at: https://www.nhlbi.nih.gov/health/educational/lose_wt/BMI/bmicalc.htm.

Alcohol and chronic alcohol use. Believe it or not, alcohol use also negatively affects the cardiovascular system and increases your risk of damage leading to dementia. You may have read reports about a glass of red wine being healthful; that's actually because of the healthful non-alcohol related compounds in the wine. But that's not what I'm referring to. We're talking about lowering your risk associated with the onset of dementia by looking at all of the risk factors. For example, as related to alcohol, did you know that alcohol is hard on the heart and circulatory system? Having more than three drinks at one time can increase your blood pressure on a temporary basis, but chronic alcohol abuse can raise it for the long term. Finally, alcohol's calorie content can result in weight gain, another risk factor for high blood pressure, diabetes, possible stroke, and the onset of dementia as a result.

Emotional health. A number of studies have linked depression to the onset of dementia. Therefore, if depression or anxiety area areas of potential concern, I strongly urge you to seek therapeutic intervention from a qualified healthcare practitioner or other counseling source.

Risk factor associated with Alzheimer's disease

Many articles separate the risks factors associated with the development of Alzheimer's disease from risks associated with the other dementias, despite Alzheimer's being a type of dementia. Risk factors associated with the development of Alzheimer's disease including but not limited to:

Gender. Women are more likely to be victimized by Alzheimer's disease than men. Some reports evidence a relationship between the onset of Alzheimer's and a decline in estrogen and progesterone due to menopause and post-menopausal physiology that is unsupported by hormone replacement. This has not been definitively proven by the medical community.

Family history of the disease. If an immediate family member (parent or sibling) has been diagnosed with Alzheimer's disease, the risk factor is reported as at least 25% higher than those individuals who do not have a biological parent or sibling who was diagnosed with dementia. In other words, the disease is more likely to present within members of the same family structure.

Genetic structure. Although familial risks discussed above might seem like they are actually genetic in nature, there are also specific genes themselves associated with the onset of Alzheimer's disease. The E-e4 (APEO-e4) gene is associated with a 20 – 25% greater risk factor of developing Alzheimer's than their peers who do not possess the gene. APE0-e4 is also thought to increase the risk of developing Alzheimer's disease at an earlier age of onset than those who do not possess the gene yet develop Alzheimer's.

There are also a variety of deterministic genes that directly cause Alzheimer's disease, which cause the onset of this disorder in approximately 5% of diagnosed cases. This is the result of genetic encoding of three specific protein structures: amyloid precursor protein (APP), presenilin-1 (PS-1), and presenilin-2 (PS-2). Of of the three, PS-1 and PS-2 are most commonly associated with early-onset Alzheimer's disease.

Other medical conditions. Other medical conditions linked to increased risk of developing Alzheimer's disease include diabetes, cardiovascular diseases. All of these types of disorders significantly impact the circulatory system, which is why the risk is so extreme as related to dementia. However, the generational nature, or the likelihood of parents raising children who develop the same disease, is a grey area. Whereas some disorders, as we'll discuss in later chapters can be prevented, especially in children; other's can only be mitigated and risks reduced. While it can be argued that some are genetically related, thus not preventable, I believe it is still possible to mitigate challenges related to these types of disorders. However, other disorders, such as Down syndrome, which is considered a high risk associated with the onset of dementia, cannot be modified, only mitigated through risk reduction strategies to prevent the the plague and tangles associated with Alzheimer's disease that typically present in the brain of many middle-aged individuals with Down's syndrome.

The goal would be to enhance circulatory related physiological processes while reducing the risks of obesity, high blood pressure, atherosclerosis, high cholesterol, and so forth.

Exposure to heavy metals. So what are heavy metals and why the huge concerns about them? Heavy metals are a group of elements belonging to what is considered the heavier molecular end of the periodic table. Although some our body needs some heavy metals in very minute amounts for healthy functioning, including copper, iron or zinc, many heavy metals are considered non-essential and are toxic to the body in excess amounts. For example, mercury, aluminum, thallium, lead, cadmium, and arsenic are considered toxic heavy metal, with mercury, lead, and arsenic the most common sources of heavy metal toxicity or poisoning.

Heavy metal toxicity, which is considered one of our risk elements here, is an excessive build-up of metals in the body. Although heavy metal toxicity is a high risk element for the onset of dementia or Alzheimer's disease specifically, heavy metal toxicity is also a general problem because the symptoms produced by heavy metal toxicity mirror many symptoms commonly found in chronic health issues, and are therefore readily dismissed by the medical community as just a problem associated with chronic illness rather than having identified the toxic source of the problem.

Although the pure traditional/allopathic medical community has generally debunked the aluminum/Alzheimer's link, to me, there is still a strong risk factor associated with the use of aluminum-based products, such as aluminum pots and pans or foil, which transfer the heavy metal into your system or foods through heat, antiperspirants transferring aluminum into your system through transdermal processes, and so forth. Eliminating or removing aluminum from your environment is a very simple option when it comes to potentially eliminating a risk factor associated with the onset of Alzheimer's disease.

You may wonder why mercury is so toxic, and how that contributes to the development of dementia? According to medical research published by Mutter et al. in the Neurology and Endocrinology Letter from October 2004 "Experimental studies have found that even smallest amounts of mercury but no other metals in low concentrations were able to cause all nerve cell changes, which are typical for Alzheimer's disease."[7] In fact, the same team published in article in a German medical journal in September 2007 that determined "Higher mercury concentrations were found in brain regions and blood of some patients with Alzheimer's disease (AD). Low levels of inorganic mercury were able to cause AD- typical nerve cell deteriorations in vitro and in animal experiments. Other metals

---

[7] Mutter, J., Naumann, J., Sadaghiani, C., Scheider, R., & Walach, H. (2004). Alzheimer disease: Mercury a pathogenic factor and apolipoprotein E as a moderator. *Neurology and Endocrinology Letter*, 25(5), 331- 339.

like zinc, aluminum, copper, cadmium, manganese, iron, and chrome are not able to elicit all of these deteriorations in low levels, yet they aggravate the toxic effects of mercury (Hg)."[8] Mercury is commonly found in many fish such as tuna, salmon, or cod. Mercury is also the primary ingredient found in amalgam (silver colored) dental fillings. As with aluminum, when exposed to heat from foods or beverages, the mercury in amalgam dental fillings leaches into your system. Therefore, mercury exposure is another modifiable risk factor. Limit your consumption of tuna or salmon (particularly canned tuna or salmon where you have both an aluminum and mercury component) unless you know the waters there are safe. For example, we get our fish oils from Norway, and our tuna and salmon are wild caught from Alaskan waters. Another modifiable method you can use to limit your mercury exposure is to have any amalgam dental filings removed, and follow with a good heavy metal detox, which is an area I work with in my naturopathic practice. To be honest, I am in the process of having my amalgams removed, and going through the detox protocol, as I write this.

Heart health. Cardiovascular disease is frequently cited as a risk factor for the onset of Alzheimer's and other dementias (as will be included below). In particular, when evidence of coronary artery disease is present including high blood pressure, stroke, diabetes, or high cholesterol, your risk of developing Alzheimer's disease increases. Therefore, steps to modify the effects, reduce the severity, and significantly limit the damage due to these disorders is pivotal not only to improve your overall health, but to limit your risk of developing Alzheimer's or one of the dementias associated with these symptoms.

---

[8]Mutter, J., Naumann, J., Scheider, R., Walach, H. (2007). Mercury and Alzheimer's disease. *Journal of Neurological Psychiatry*, 75(9), 528 – 538.

Chapter Four: Healthy child, healthy adult, healthy senior: Breaking the generational dementia curse

Looking at the risk factors for dementia detailed in the previous chapter of this book, you can easily see how failure to reduce the risk of one factor, such as heart disease, can easily lead to a cascade of other risk factors ranging from high cholesterol to high blood pressure.

The important thing here is to recognize that each of these factors have a high element of increased risk of heredity from one generation to the next. If a parent has high cholesterol or high blood pressure, it is highly likely that the next generation will suffer from the same malady *even if not genetically predisposed.*

In other words, where we might have a genetic predisposed risk for various illnesses, such as breast or ovarian cancer if you are positive for the BRAC-2 gene, the increased risk of contracting these disorders cannot be eliminated. No matter what efforts you take to mitigate the risk of contracting breast cancer if you are BRAC-2 positive, there will ALWAYS be some element of increased risk.

The same is true for the APEO-e4 gene and risk of Alzheimer's disease; you cannot eliminate the risk due to being genetically predisposed, *however, based on mitigating other risk factors, you CAN significantly reduce the genetically predisposed risk of developing the dementia.*

Remember: for those without the APEO-e4 gene (genetic predisposition), if an immediate family member (parent or sibling) has been diagnosed with Alzheimer's disease, the risk factor is reported as

at least 25% higher than those individuals who do not have a biological parent or sibling who was diagnosed with dementia, and that's on top of the 25% increased risk we already know is present within members of the same family structure. But remember, there are other factors in addition to the APEO-e4 gene that contribute to the onset of dementia, and the certainty one associates with heredity can be minimized or eliminated.
Certainty of the onset of dementia need not be the case! You can break the cycle! You can break the generational curse of dementia.

Remember we said: Not counting all other forms of dementia Alzheimer's disease alone currently affects 5.5 million people in the US, with an anticipated rise to 16 million by the year 2050. If more people focused on prevention, whether as an adult, and especially by instilling healthy habits in children that are maintained into adulthood, even now with 33 years to go until 2050, I believe that total number of individuals diagnosed with Alzheimer's disease in the US would be dramatically less than 16 million people! And given that Alzheimer's disease is the most frequently diagnosed type of dementia, and the fact that other dementias share most of the same risk factors, I believe this is very significant and can easily be achieved!

You may argue and say, what do the children have to do with it? Most of the risk factors identified in the previous chapter are diagnosed when individuals are in their middle-aged adult years, right? For example, type 2 diabetes, high blood pressure, and high cholesterol are only diagnosed in adults, right?

Sadly, the answer to that is a resounding NO!!! These issues, as well as the other risk elements are no longer limited to middle-aged or older adults! More and more of these risk elements associated with the onset of dementia are being diagnosed in children! And it is frightening! The medical community is baffled yet does not address the central issue or the long tem consequences, such as dementia or Alzheimer's disease when talking to parents of children.

Look at a snapshot of some statistics:

- Among children ages 3 to 18 years, 3.4% have pre-hypertension and 3.6% have hypertension; this is even higher in middle-school and high-school athletes where almost 15% of the student-athletes have high blood pressure;

- In adolescents who are obese, more than 30% of boys and between 23 -- 30% percent of girls have pre-hypertension or hypertension;

- One out of every five (20%) young children or teens have unhealthy cholesterol levels;

- The prevalence of Type 2 diabetes among those ages 10 to 19 rose 30% in the last decade. Most children who develop type 2 diabetes have a family member with type 2 diabetes; 45–80% have a parent with type 2 diabetes, and 74–90% report at least one affected first- or second-degree relative;

- Upwards of 15–20% (5 million adolescents) of America's teens aged 12–18 years are overweight;

- An average of 3,800 children under the age of 18 try smoking for the first time every day. Of those, 2,100 youth will become daily smokers, creating over 766,500 new teen smokers every year;

- Teens who start smoking become addicted faster than adults, and it takes less nicotine to addict a teen smoker than it does an adult.

- By age 15, about one third of all teens have had at least 1 drink, increasing to 60% by the time a teen turns 18 years of age;

- People ages 12 through 20 drink 11% of all alcohol consumed in the United States, typically drinking more than adults due to binge drinking in one sitting;

- 5.1 million young people reported binge drinking (for males 5 or more drinks and for females 4 or more drinks on the same occasion within a few hours) at least once in the past month, with 1.3 million young people reported binge drinking on 5 or more days over the past month;

- Binge drinking by for the pre-teen age group between 9–13 is roughly 3 drinks, ages 14–15, binge drinking increases to about 4 drinks, and by ages 16–17 binge drinking consumption increases to about 5 drinks per sitting.

Given our concerns about risks associated with the onset of dementia although we discussed the issues related to alcohol consumption in the previous chapter, for children it is even worse! Anatomically and physiologically, young people's brains keep developing well into their 20s. Alcohol can alter this development, potentially affecting both brain structure and function. This may cause cognitive or learning problems and/or make the brain more prone to alcohol dependence. This is especially a risk when people start drinking young and drink heavily. In addition to contributing to the other risks of alcohol consumption, such as diabetes and obesity, this structural damage itself can create an early risk element for the onset of dementia later in life. It's a setup for the perfect storm.

Other risks developing in childhood create the same concerns. For example, atherosclerosis can actually begin in childhood, progress slowly and appear so mild that most doctors don't identify a problem until the child matures and becomes a young adult who suffers a stroke. One of the biggest modifiable risk factors associated with childhood atherosclerosis is childhood obesity.

High blood pressure is becoming more common in children as well, particularly due to the increasing rates associated with childhood obesity. However, like atherosclerosis, diagnosing high blood pressure in children is not as routine an occurrence or process as it is for adults. It is not something pediatrician or other doctors typically look for in children. Additionally, whereas for adults, figures associated with high blood pressure diagnosis are pretty clear cut, with the ideal blood pressure reading at 120/80 mm Hg; for children assessing normal blood pressure levels is age, sex, and height dependent.

High cholesterol is also a growing concern for children, which like high blood pressure is becoming more common with the increase in childhood obesity rates. The American Academy of Pediatrics recommends that all children should be screened once between ages 9 and 11, and again between ages 17 and 21. However, selective screening is also recommended for children with a family history of high cholesterol, or for children with a BMI greater than the 95th percentile on charts for children aged 2-8 years of age, or the 85th percentile for children aged 12 – 16 years when other risk factors are present, such as diabetes, high blood pressure, or exposure to cigarette smoke. When these risk factors are present in the home, the first screening is recommended when the child is 2 years of age. The problem is, like atherosclerosis or high blood pressure, routine questions regarding risk factors are not often asked when a child sees a pediatrician, and diagnosis is not as simple in children as it is in adults. Therefore, these are often areas in childhood health screenings that should be, but are not always assessed. Attention to these areas is particularly important however, when looking to proactively mitigate risk associated with the development of dementia when the individual is still a young child.

Type 2 diabetes has actually been described in the medical literature as a new epidemic in the American pediatric population. As recently as just 25 years ago, in 1992, it was rare for most pediatric centers to have patients with type 2 diabetes. By 1994, type 2 diabetes accounted for up to 16% of new cases of pediatric diabetes in urban areas, and by 1999, it accounted for between 8–45% of newly diagnosed pediatric cases of type 2 diabetes, depending on geographic location. In fact, type 2 diabetes is not the only problem, type 1 diabetes has also increased upwards of 21% in the pediatric population.

Most children who develop type 2 diabetes have a family member with type 2 diabetes; 45–80% have a parent with type 2 diabetes, and 74–90% report at least one affected first- or second-degree relative. Risk factors include puberty, intrauterine exposure to diabetes, sedentary lifestyle, and female gender. Additionally, childhood type-2 diabetes is more likely to occur in children and teens who are inactive. With the sharp rise in computer games and TV-watching and the trend toward abandoning physical education in schools, fewer children are participating in sports. Once type 2 diabetes is diagnosed in a child, the persistence of obesity interferes with the response to treatment and exacerbates the risk of also developing high cholesterol high blood pressure, and, atherosclerosis.

The root of many of these childhood disorders, or at least a major risk factor associated with obesity, which statistics above highlighted are increasing dramatically, as are statistics for other risk factors – coincidence? Not at all, there is a direct relationship between childhood obesity and other risk factors we've discussed in this chapter. And sadly, in the long term, childhood obesity also is associated with having obesity as an adult.

So, what are some of the risk factors that contribute to childhood obesity? Diet is a primary consideration, for example, more children are being fed diets higher fat and simple sugars rather than healthier fruits and vegetables, while simultaneously becoming more sedentary watching television or playing games on the computer as opposed to physically exercising where more calories are expended. Second, the increased rated of obesity in children is also witnessed by an increased rate of obesity in adults. What's happened? Children of obese parents are more likely to be overweight themselves. Parental obesity may also reflect a family environment that promotes excess eating and insufficient activity. Yes, there is a potential genetic component leading overweight parents to have children who are overweight, however - even children with genetic risk for overweight will still only become overweight if they consume more calories than they use. You can mitigate genetic predispositions, remember? However, genetic or not, parents with poor nutritional habits and who lead sedentary lifestyles role model these behaviors for their children, thereby creating an "obesigenic" home environment.

Depressive and bipolar disorders are not just emotional issues some children and teens suffer from. As relates to our discussion of risk factors associated with the onset of dementia, most notably those relating to cardiovascular and circulatory health, there is current medical evidence that major depression and bipolar disorder in adolescents are associated with an increased risk of early cardiovascular disease.

Statistics at the beginning of this chapter on childhood cigarette smoking were dramatic. However, what the number of children and teens smoking does not tell you is that smoking and exposure to smoking increases the risk of developing early cardiovascular disease. Children/teenagers who smoke themselves are likely to continue smoking into adulthood, thus increasing their risk of early cardiovascular and circulatory diseases even more than those who start smoking as adults.

SPECIAL NOTE: Although each of these risk factors affecting children can take up entire text books on presentation, diagnosis, assessments, other health risks associated with and affecting each, treatment plans, prognosis, and so forth, this chapter was only meant to provide the highlights of the various risk factors affecting children that contribute to the development of dementia. Therefore, it may seem rather limited in scope, but every effort was made to maintain the focus of this book. Should you wish to discuss any of these risk factors in greater detail, I am always available to do so!

This chapter has discussed the risk factors associated with the onset of dementia in terms of affecting children and teens in rapidly increasing rates, thus automatically predisposing children to dementia much earlier in the developmental cycle than one might have original thought. In other words, while we think of dementia as a disease complex affecting older individuals, especially Alzheimer's disease, in more and more cases, the development of risk factors leading to dementia are beginning in childhood rather than adulthood. The statistics and diagnoses concerns presented here speak for themselves.

Therefore, we can ask ourselves, is the increase in cases of dementia and more specifically Alzheimer's disease due to children becoming predisposed to the disorder due to developing risk factors in their youth rather than in their adult years as was previously, almost exclusively the case? I strongly believe the answer to this is yes, the statistical rise of Alzheimer's disease and other forms of dementia anticipated by the year 2050 is due to the increase in childhood risk factors contributing to a life long developmental process of the disease.

If this is the case, then the next question I will ask you is: If we address childhood risk factors associated with the onset of dementia, can we mitigate the risk of that child developing dementia in their later adult years? The answer is YES!

Addressing the risk factors associated with the onset of dementia affecting the adult population can mitigate risk for the individual as an adult. But that doesn't break the familial cycle of one generation developing dementia and seemingly passing that predisposition on to the next generation, who then passes it on to the next, and so on. If you break the cycle while the individual is a child by addressing risk factors early, there is less likelihood of these risk factors continuing into their adult years, and a significantly lower likelihood of becoming victimized by dementia, and a parallel significantly reduction in the risk factors perpetuating throughout the generations.

Chapter Five: Traditional pharmacological interventions and side effects

In the last chapter we talked about risk factors. If you go to your doctor, they are likely to write a prescription for a pharmaceutical agent that will alter your physiology to mediate the issue - in other words, it will try to lessen symptoms or make the problem go away. For chronic health issues, such as diabetes, usually the pharmaceutical will only lessen symptoms and the problem remains; if the pharmaceutical is no longer used, symptoms typically return. Additionally, pharmacological agents themselves usually carry with them potential negative side effects.

Now, this might separate me from a lot of other naturopaths and even individuals seeking only natural remedies, but I want to make this blanket statement up front. *I believe there is a need for pharmaceutical intervention in a limited number of situations*:

1. As a temporary crutch to get you over a physical or emotional hurdle before a natural remedy can be taken or become effective;
2. For some health challenges where the individual body does not react to natural remedies;
3. When only a pharmaceutical agent is available as a remedy for your particular health challenge.

So you see, I am not against pharmaceuticals. They have their proper time and place in our lives. However, I also believe if you are going to take a pharmaceutical, you need to know the risks associated with that pharmaceutical. Just as we're talking about risks associated with dementia, there are additional risks in the dementia risk mitigation plan when treating with pharmaceuticals. Helping you be an informed consumer is what this chapter is all about!

I also want to start out this chapter with a disclaimer: there are thousands and thousands of pharmaceutical agents available in the marketplace. Based on the numbers alone, it would be virtually impossible to discuss each of them independently within the limited space of this chapter. Therefore, when mentioned by name, those drugs, are representative of the general grouping of medications available for a specific health risk.

So let's talk about pharmaceuticals and the idea of using specific pharmaceuticals to mitigate the risks discussed in the last chapter.

Gender. Yes, it is true that women are more likely to be victimized by Alzheimer's disease than men due to hormone challenges as a woman ages. However, to date there are no reports that pharmacological supplementation with any of the over 50 combinations of estrogen and progesterone available in hormone replacement therapies, not including the various numbers of estrogen or progesterone only pharmaceuticals, demonstrating this reduces the gender-based risk associated with the onset of dementia. And remember, even standard hormone replacement therapy for women (and men) carries risks ranging from blood clots to cancer and must be considered in any decision you make regarding your hormonal health.

Genetic structure. Although presence of the E-e4 (APEO-e4) gene is associated with a 20 – 25% greater risk factor of developing Alzheimer's disease, or for the encoding of the genetic encoding of the three protein structures (amyloid precursor protein (APP), presenilin-1 (PS-1), and presenilin-2 (PS-2), there are no pharmaceutical agents currently available that will correct for this particular genetic abnormality. As more research into genetic pharmacology is performed, perhaps this will come to pass. But I suspect that as is the case with many other pharmaceuticals, for example one I know of for a particular type of leukemia, the pharmaceutical only corrects the genetic abnormality itself, it will not correct for the underlying diagnosis. Thus if an agent was developed, it would be more likely to address the genetic protein encoding dysfunction as opposed to the genetic risk based on E-e4 (APEO-e4). Therefore, I personally believe, despite advances in pharmacology, that this is and will remain unmodifiable.

Heavy metals. One of the lesser acknowledged but non-the-less serious risk factors is exposure to heavy metals. These were discussed at length in a previous chapter, but in this chapter we're going to discuss the pharmacological avenues to remove heavy metals and the potential risk involved.

One of the terms often used in medical circles regarding the removal of heavy metals in your system is through a process called chelation. Chelation is a process where toxic metal ions are bound to other molecules, and in the attached state, removed from the body.

However, many chelation agents only work with specific heavy metals; and some heavy metals cannot be removed through chelation.

There are several primary pharmaceutical chelation agents, two of which will be mentioned here just to give you an idea of how dangerous these can be. For example, Dimercaprol (also known as British Anti-Lewisite or BAL), is used as a chelation agent for the treatment of arsenic or mercury. In this case, this pharmaceutical is administered via injection. However, potential negative side effects can include a sensation of tightness in the chest, abdomen, limbs, or chest, hypertension, tachycardia, nausea and vomiting, pain or even abscesses at the injection site, tremors, conjunctivitis, nasal discharge, paresthesia in the hands, and can be toxic to the kidneys! Additionally, this agent is based in peanut oil, so it is not appropriate for those with nut or bean allergies. Additionally, if the patient has issues with iron, cadmium or selenium, this can form additional toxic complexes in the body.

The other we'll discuss here is called Penicillamine (please don't get confused, although this is metabolite of penicillin, this was not a typo), but is also known by the names Cuprimine and Depen and is orally administered either in capsule or tablet form. Typically, this pharmaceutical agent is used for arsenic poisoning, but can also be used for mercury, copper, or lead poisoning. Particularly as our reason for examining pharmaceutical chelation agents is to reduce the risk of dementia, this particular agent is known to actually worsen or even create the development of neurological symptoms in patients, causes diarrhea, alters taste, can cause a rash, proteinuria, and leukopenia, not to mention nausea and vomiting, fevers, loss of appetite, neuropathies, renal failure, hepatitis, pancreatitis, and hemolytic anemia. Of course, as a metabolite of penicillin, this cannot be used by individuals with penicillin allergies.

Heart health. As discussed in the last chapter, cardiovascular disease is frequently cited as a risk factor for the onset of Alzheimer's and other dementias and often presents as high blood pressure, stroke, diabetes, or high cholesterol, your risk of developing Alzheimer's disease increases. But what is the typical approach to treating these conditions? Obviously, pharmaceuticals. Let's examine some of the options.

A plethora of pharmaceuticals are available to treat *high blood pressure*, classified into a number of drug types and classes to address multiple mitigation strategies and thus reduce high blood pressure. For example, angiotensin II converting enzymes, or ACE, inhibitors are commonly prescribed to reduce the muscle tension and enlarge or dilate within arteries and thus reduce blood pressure. Some of the more common ACE inhibitors that you may either be prescribed or be familiar with by name include: enalapril (Vasotec), captopril (Capoten), lisinopril (Zesril and Prinvil), benazepril (Lotensin), quinapril (Accupril), perindopril (Aceon), ramipril (Altace), trandolapril (Mavik), fosinopril (Monopril), and moexipril (Univasc). Common side effects from ACE inhibitors in general include cough, hypotension (or low blood pressure), fatigue, and headache. Sadly, the list of common side effects offered by most pharmaceutical companies do not include issues related to other side effects, such as nutrient depletion. For example, lisinopril depletes zinc, which is necessary for a wide variety of health needs, including healthy immune function, skin health and hair growth, metabolism of food and absorption of other nutrients, the ability to maintain a proper hormone balance, digestive health, maintaining mental clarity, promoting wound healing, required for proper DNA synthesis, and more!

Another class of pharmaceuticals to treat high blood pressure are angiotensin II receptor blockers (ARBs) and like the type name implies, block angiotensin II from binding to their receptors on muscles surrounding blood vessels, enabling blood vessels to enlarge and dilate, thereby lowering blood pressure. Whereas the previous classification, ACE inhibitors prevented the formation of angiotensin II, this type blocks binding. Some of the more common ARBs that you may either be prescribed or be familiar with by name include: losartan (Cozaar), irbesartan (Avapro), valsartan (Diovan), candesartan (Atacand), olmesartan (Benicar), telmisartan (Micardis), eprosartan

(Teveten), and azilsartan (Edarbi). As you can imagine, angiotensin II receptor blockers have their own list of common side effects, including cough, low blood pressure, fatigue, headache, indigestion, diarrhea, and increased levels of potassium.

Still another class of blood pressure pharmaceuticals are called beta-blockers, which block norepinephrine and adrenaline from binding to specific receptors on the organs and muscles throughout the body, which of course includes the muscles surrounding blood vessels, causing them to narrow. Like other blood pressure reducing pharmaceuticals, beta blockers dilate blood vessels and thus reduce blood pressure. Some of the more common ARBs that you may either be prescribed or be familiar with by name include: acebutolol (Sectral), atenolol (Tenormin), bisoprolol fumarate (Zebeta), carvedilol(Coreg), esmolol (Brevibloc), meoprolol (Lopressor, Toprol XL), nadolol (Cogard), nebivolol (Bystolic), and propranolol (Hemaneol, Indeal, LA Inderal XL, InnoPran XL). Common side effects of beta blockers include: fatigue, dizziness, shortness of breath, impotence, and low blood pressure.

In addition to beta-blockers, another type of pharmaceutical is called a calcium channel blocker. Essentially, all muscle cells in our body require calcium which are used throughout the body to allow the actual muscle cells to contract. Calcium channel blockers prevent calcium from entering muscle cells, thereby preventing muscles around blood vessels (along with the muscles around the heart) from contracting and raising blood pressure. Thus, calcium channel blockers relax muscle cells and thus lower blood pressure. calcium is needed by all muscle cells, including those of the heart and muscles and surrounding arteries, in order for the cells to contract. CCBs inhibit the movement of calcium into muscle cells.

There are three major types of calcium channel blockers on the market: dihydropyridines. Some of the more common calcium channel blockers that you may either be prescribed or be familiar with by name include a group of pharmaceuticals with amlodipine (Norvasc) alone, or in combination with another medication, such as amlodipine and atorvastatin, a cholesterol lowering drug, is Caduet. There are also another two types of calcium channel blockers referred to as non-dihydropyridine agents. One type is verapamil (Calan, Covera, Isoptin, and Verelan), and the other is diltiazem (Cardizem, Tiazac, Dilacor, and Diltia). Amlodipine and benazepril, an ACE inhibitor, is known as Lotrel. Amlodipine and valsartan (an AFB) are known by the name Exforge. These are just examples of what is available as some pharmaceuticals designed to lower blood pressure belong to multiple groups and work through multiple pathways and mechanisms to lower blood pressure. Common side effects of calcium channel blockers include water retention and swelling in the arms and legs, shortness of breath, headache, rash, and constipation.

Diuretics are among the oldest known medications for treating high blood pressure. Essentially, the role of a diuretic is to remove salt from the body through pharmacological action on the kidneys. Removing salt is thought to relax muscles surrounding blood vessels, and thus lower blood pressure. Typically, blood pressure meds in this class are used in conjunction with pharmaceuticals from other types to combine their mechanisms of action in lowering blood pressure and increase the effectiveness of the non-diuretic drug. Some of the most commonly used diuretics include hydrochlorothiazide (Hydrodiuril), chlorthalidone, and loop dieretics called furosemide (Lasix), buetanide (Bumex), and torsemide (Demadex). Another form is called Dyazide, which is the combination of triamterene and hydrochlorothiazide. However, common side effects of diuretics include low blood pressure, low blood potassium levels, dehydration, fatigue, increased uric acid levels, and increased blood blood glucose levels, which can be particularly dangerous for those who are pre-diabetic or diabetic. It is important to know that hydrochlorothiazide can also increases homocysteine levels, a significant risk for the development of atherosclerosis and cardiac health, the very disorders we're trying to mitigate as related to dementia.

Alpha-blockers are similar to beta blockers, in that the pharmaceuticals in this category act on the muscles surrounding blood vessels which have not only beta receptors, but alpha receptors as well. When alpha receptors are stimulated, like stimulation of beta receptors, the muscles surrounding the arteries contract and narrow the arteries and thus increase the pressure related to arterial blood flow, increasing blood pressure. By blocking the alpha receptor, alpha-blockers relax the muscles and lower blood pressure. Some of the more common alpha blockers include terazosin (Hytrin) and doxazosin (Cardura). Common negative side effects include nausea weakness, dizziness and vertigo, and low blood pressure.

Alpha-beta blockers are another type of pharmaceutical to lower blood pressure, and work the same way as alpha-blockers but also slow the heartbeat at the same time. As a result, less blood is pumped through the vessels, vessels dilate and blood pressure is lowered. Two of the more common alpha-beta blockers are carvedilol (Coreg) and labetalol (Trandate). Like their blood pressure pharmaceuticals from other categories, Alpha-beta blockers are not without their negative side effects, including fatigue, slow heart rate, shortness of breath, dizziness and vertigo, weight gain, and low blood pressure.

Finally, minoxidil can be used to lower blood pressure. This may surprise you as most people associate minoxidil as a remedy for male pattern baldness, but it also dilates blood vessels. As discussed with other classes of pharmaceuticals, when blood vessels can dilate, blood pressure is reduced. However, minoxidil is not without its negative side effects as well. For example, patients report swelling throughout the body, weight gain, headaches, and increased heart rates.

Diabetes:

One report that I recently read stated there are in excess of 157 different medications for diabetes; and that's just for type 2, which is what I will be discussing here in our presentation on risk factors associated with the onset of dementia. Given the majority of these 157 pharmaceuticals are oral drugs, those requiring injections are excluded from our presentation in this chapter.

Like all of the other pharmaceuticals prescribed for risk factors associated with dementia, those for type 2 diabetes also fall into varied classes and types based on their mechanism of action.

Alpha-glucosidase inhibitors help your body break down starchy foods and table sugar. Rather than letting the body break down starches that will immediately increase your blood glucose level, by inhibiting the breakdown the release of glucose into the blood is slowed, and thus lowers the body's blood sugar level. Common alpha-glucosidase inhibitors include: acarbose (Precose), and miglitol (Glyset). The majority of the common negative side effects are associated with digestive discomfort, including nausea, gas, and bloating.

Another class of pharmaceuticals targeting type 2 diabetes are the biguanides, which decrease how much sugar your liver makes, decrease how much sugar your intestines absorb, make your body more sensitive to insulin, and help your muscles absorb glucose. The most common biguanide is metformin (Glucophage, Metformin

Hydrochloride ER, Glumetza, Riomet, and Fortamet). As with alpha-glucosidase inhibitors, the most common negative side effects from biguanides affect the digestive tract, including nausea, gas, and bloating. Additionally, patients report a difference in their ability to taste various foods. Other negative side effects include metallic taste in the mouth and diarrhea.

As one of the most common pharmaceuticals targeting diabetes, similar to drugs for high blood pressure or to lower cholesterol, metformin can also be combined with other drugs for type 2 diabetes that significantly increase the mechanisms of action to lower blood glucose levels. Some of the common combination drugs include: metformin-alogliptin (Kazano), metformin-canagliflozin (Invokamet), metformin-dapagliflozin (Xigduo XR), metformin-empagliflozin (Synjardy), metformin-glipizide (Metaglip), metformin-glyburide (Glucovance), metformin-linagliptin (Jentadueto), metformin-pioglitazone (Actoplus), metformin-repaglinide (PrandiMet), metformin-rosiglitazone (Avandamet), metformin-saxagliptin (Kombiglyze XR), and metformin-sitagliptin (Janumet). You'll see similar combinations in some of the other categories below.

There is only one pharmaceutical on the marketing in the United States to treat type 2 diabetes referred to as a dopamine agonist; bromocriptine (Parlodel). It's not known exactly how this drug works to treat type 2 diabetes. However, the theorized mechanism of action to explain how it lowers blood sugar is that the pharmaceutical may affect the natural rhythms in your body and prevent insulin resistance.

Another class of pharmaceuticals to treat type 2 diabetes are known as DPP-4 inhibitors which help the body continue to make insulin. Essentially, DPP-4 inhibitors work by inhibiting the action of an enzyme in the body that leads to an increase in the release of insulin, and it simultaneously decreases the production of glucose by the liver. This combination essentially forces the pancreas to make more insulin. They work by reducing blood sugar without causing hypoglycemia (low blood sugar), which is a common side effect of many pharmaceuticals prescribed to treat type 2 diabetes. Some of the more common pharmaceuticals in this class include: alogliptin (Nesina), alogliptin-metformin (Kazano), alogliptin-pioglitazone (Oseni), linagliptin (Tradjenta), linagliptin-empagliflozin (Glyxambi), linagliptin-metformin (Jentadueto), saxagliptin (Onglyza), saxagliptin-metformin (Kombiglyze XR), sitagliptin (Januvia), sitagliptin-metformin (Janumet and Janumet XR), and sitagliptin and simvastatin (Juvisync). Common negative side effects include digestive distress, as with the other pharmaceuticals used to treat type 2 diabetes, but in particular, sitagliptin (Januvia) is reported as causing serious allergic reactions, sore throat, upper respiratory infection, and headache.

Glucagon-like peptides (incretin mimetics) are similar to the natural hormone called incretin. Essentially glucagon-like peptides work to increase B-cell growth and how much insulin your body uses. They also decrease your appetite and how much glucagon your body uses while simultaneously slowing the rate at which your stomach empties, maintaining a full or satiated feeling longer. Common pharmaceuticals in this class include: albiglutide (Tanzeum); dulaglutide (Trulicity); exenatide (Byetta); exenatide extended-release (Bydureon); and liraglutide (Victoza).

Another category of pharmaceuticals to treat type 2 diabetes are the Meglitinides. Meglitinides help your body release insulin by stimulating the release of more insulin from beta cells. Common medications in this category include: nateglinide (Starlix); repaglinide (Prandin); and repaglinide-metformin (Prandimet). Common negative side effects of meglitinides include problems associated with hypoglycemia (low blood glucose levels), fatigue, dizziness, and weight gain.

Yet another class of pharmaceuticals to treat type 2 diabetes are referred to as sodium glucose transporter (SGLT) 2 inhibitors which work by preventing the kidneys from retaining glucose. Instead, these drugs foster the release of glucose through the urinary tract. Common SGLT 2 inhibitors include: dapagliflozin (Farxiga), dapagliflozin-metformin (Xigduo XR), canagliflozin (Invokana), canagliflozin-metformin (Invokamet), empagliflozin (Jardiance), empagliflozin-linagliptin (Glyxambi), and empagliflozin-metformin (Synjardy).

Sulfonylureas are among the oldest orally administered drugs used to treat type 2 diabetes on the market today. Sulfonylureas work by stimulating the pancreas to produce more insulin with the help of beta cells, thus causing the body to actually increase it's own production of insulin. Common sulfonylureas include: glimepiride (Amaryl), glimepiride-pioglitazone (Duetact), glimeperide-rosiglitazone (Avandaryl), glipizide (Glucotrol), glipizide-metformin (Metaglip), glyburide (DiaBeta, Glynase, Micronase), glyburide-metformin (Glucovance), chlorpropamide (Diabinese), tolazamide (Tolinase), and tolbutamide (Orinase, Tol-Tab). One of the primary negative side effects of solfonylureas is the significantly increased potential for hypoglycemia (low blood sugar). Other common negative side effects of sulfonylureas include: skin rash or itching, sensitivity to sunlight, upset stomach, and weight gain.

Yet another classification of pharmaceuticals to treat type 2 diabetes are thiazolidinediones which work by decreasing the level of glucose in your liver while simultaneously helping fat cells to optimize their insulin use. Common pharmaceuticals in this class that you may have heard about on television or see in magazine advertising include:

rosiglitazone (Avandia), rosiglitazone-glimepiride (Avandaryl), rosiglitizone-metformin (Amaryl M), pioglitazone (Actos), pioglitazone-alogliptin (Oseni), pioglitazone-glimepiride (Duetact), and pioglitazone-metformin (Actoplus Met, Actoplus Met XR). Risks of negative side effects with pharmaceuticals in this class are particularly troublesome, and very important to our discussion as reducing risk related to the onset of dementia as the use of thiazolidinediones come with a significantly increased risk of developing heart disease should not be used in patients with symptoms of heart failure. Additionally, it is recommended that liver enzymes should be checked regularly with use. Other negative side effects commonly reported include weight gain, fatigue, swelling of the legs or ankles, and increased risk for fractures in female patients.

Many individuals who are prescribed medication to treat type 2 diabetes are also prescribed medication for many other medical issues. It is critical to note that in particular, those individuals who are prescribed pharmaceuticals to treat type 2 diabetes consult their pharmacist if they are also prescribed any type of prescription or over the counter medications due to the potential to adversely interact with one or more of the drugs prescribed. These include but are not limited to some: heart medications, decongestants, antibiotics, thiazides, steroids, thyroid drugs, estrogens, oral contraceptives, seizure medications, psychiatric medications, and cholesterol medications. Additionally, digestive enzyme medications (such as amylase, pancreatin) may reduce the effectiveness of alpha-glucosidase inhibitors and should not be taken at the same time. Sulfonylureas may increase the risk of death from cardiovascular disease. Prolonged exercise and alcohol intake increase the risk for hypoglycemia. Patients undergoing surgery or who have had recent trauma, stress, or infection may need to switch from a sulfonylurea to insulin to manage blood sugar levels. People with kidney or liver disease in particular need to be very cautious taking many of the commonly prescribed medications for type 2 diabetes.

Other serious warnings related to the use of pharmaceuticals used to treat type 2 diabetes that are class or drug specific include the risk for thiazolidinediones, which may cause or exacerbate heart failure. Trouble breathing, rapid weight gain and fluid retention may indicate the onset of heart failure. Avandia may potentially increase the risk of heart attack. Alpha-glucosidase inhibitors should not be used in people with intestinal diseases such as inflammatory bowel disease or intestinal obstruction. People with a history of liver disease, heavy drinking, or kidney disease may not be able to take biguanides. Inform medical personnel of biguanide use prior to any radiological tests which require injection of dye. Severe hypersensitivity reactions have occurred during use of sitagliptin.

High cholesterol. As widespread as these issues are in our society, it should be no surprise that there are in excess of 30 different pharmaceutical agents typically prescribed to reduce cholesterol. While pharmaceuticals to lower cholesterol also fall into a number of categories, the goal of all are the same: to decrease your low-density lipoprotein (LDL) cholesterol, the "bad" cholesterol that increases the risk of heart disease, to decrease your triglycerides, a type of fat in the blood that also increases the risk of heart disease, and to increase your high-density lipoprotein (HDL) cholesterol, the "good" cholesterol that offers protection from heart disease.

The first type of pharmaceutical most people are placed on when diagnosed with high cholesterol is a statin. Some of the more common statins available include: Altoprev (lovastatin), Crestor (rosuvastatin), Lescol (fluvastatin), Lipitor (atorvastatin), Livalo (pitavastatin), Pravachol (pravastatin), and Zocor (simvastatin). Possible negative side effects however, include constipation, nausea, diarrhea, stomach pain, cramps, muscle soreness, pain and weakness. Like medications to lower blood pressure, these drugs are also affected by consuming grapefruit juice. While statins have their place as the mainstay of cholesterol reducing drugs, statins seriously rob the body of CoQ10. Essentially, the way statins work is all in the liver, where the creation of cholesterol is blocked. However, while the enzyme within the liver to create cholesterol is blocked, it is also blocking the pathway where CoQ10 is created. As CoQ10 is responsible for energy production and cell functioning, that's why many people taking statins to control their cholesterol levels will feel fatigued and suffer from other health issues due to poor cellular performance and functioning throughout every cell in their body! Other nutrient deficiencies from statins include selenium, copper, vitamin E, and zinc.

Bile acid binding resins are another type of cholesterol lowering medication that are used to decrease LDL cholesterol. Essentially, bile acid resins bind to bile acids within the intestines. This action prevents the bile acids from being reabsorbed into the bloodstream from the intestines. With a shortage of cholesterol coming from the intestine into the liver, the body still needs to produce cholesterol, it uses already in the blood, thus reducing the amount of LDL cholesterol circulating in the body. Typically, bile acid binding resins are used by people who cannot take statins. Common pharmaceuticals in this category include Colestid (colestipol), Prevalite (cholestyramine), and Welchol (colesevelam). Common negative side effects from these medications include constipation, bloating, nausea, and gas.

Another category in is the cholesterol absorption inhibitor, obviously as the name implies, it inhibits the absorption of cholesterol rather than inhibits its production. The most common pharmaceutical in this category, also used to decrease LDL cholesterol, and to a lesser extent, simultaneously increase HDL cholesterol and decease triglyceride levels, is Zetia (ezetimibe). However, common negative side effects include stomach pain, fatigue, and muscle soreness.

Another classification of cholesterol lowering medication combines cholesterol absorption inhibitors and statins, the most common of which is Vytorin (ezetimibe-simvastatin), which also works to decrease LDL and triglyceride levels while increasing HDL cholesterol. Unfortunately, possible negative side effects include the combination of side effects from both categories, including but not limited to stomach pain, fatigue, gas, constipation, abdominal pain, cramps, muscle soreness, pain and weakness. As is the case for statins alone, there is an interaction when consumed with grapefruit juice.

Combination statin and calcium channel blockers are often prescribed for those who have both high cholesterol and high blood pressure. For example, the drug Caduet (atorvastatin-amlodipine) decreases LDL cholesterol and triglycerides while lowering blood pressure. However, common side effects from the combination of these include a myriad of other symptoms, including facial and neck flushing, dizziness, heart palpitations, muscle pain and weakness. Like statins alone, there are problems associated with grapefruit juice consumption.

Healthy lifestyle. In a previous chapter we mentioned that healthier lifestyles typically include suggestions including reduce the risks of coronary heart disease or diabetes through not only a healthy diet, but through smoking cessation, minimal alcohol consumption, and weight loss. And guess what? There are pharmaceuticals available to help you achieve your goals; but like all the drugs discussed so far, pharmaceuticals in this category can also be problematic and are not without their own risks.

Smoking cessation. While nicotine patches and chewing gum have their own issues, prescriptions are no longer needed to obtain them, therefore they will not be included in this section. However, there are two specific pharmaceuticals that are non-nicotine based that are frequently prescribed for smoking cessation to reduce or eliminate tobacco cravings, aid with symptoms of tobacco withdrawal, and help prevent relapse. The first pharmaceutical is bupropion (Zyban), which is also prescribed as a remedy for depression. Although physicians prescribe the drug, and certainly the pharmaceutical companies sell and have FDA approval for the use of bupropion for smoking cessation, pharmacologists have no clear understanding of the specific mechanisms of action for this drug in relation to smoking cessation, other than to claim it works. Common side effects include potential changes in mood and behavior including anger, agitation, thoughts or attempts at suicide, and depressed mood, and insomnia or other sleep disturbances.

Varenicline (Chantix) is the other pharmaceutical for smoking cessation that helps to reduce the craving for nicotine, and lessens withdrawal symptoms, by working in the brain to reduce the physical effects of nicotine. This also means that if you quit, and then feel the need to smoke again, or relapse, that you will not get as much pleasure from it when using Chantix. Common negative side effects include headaches, insomnia and sleep disturbances including strange dreams, digestive issues including constipation, intestinal gas, nausea, and changes in taste, and depression including thoughts of an attempted suicide. While these side effects are troublesome, yes, the benefits of smoking cessation are important for a wide variety of reasons. However, our discussion remains focused on smoking cessation as part of an overall program to prevent dementia and cardiovascular disease. However, varenicline actually increases the risk of stroke and heart attack. If you are working to reduce the risks associated with the onset of dementia and wish to embark on a pharmaceutically-based smoking cessation program, I strongly advice you look into other options than varenicline.

Weight loss. One might think that a healthy lifestyle should include healthy eating plans to achieve weight loss. However, in addition to the plethora of over the counter weight loss aids, there are over 20 different pharmaceuticals widely prescribed for weight loss. As has been the case for other medication needs, such as high blood pressure or high cholesterol, there are different categories of weight loss drugs as well. For example, some are appetite suppressants, others work on the brain and appetite satiation centers. In fact, that full feeling is related to numerous physiological processes. For example, when you feel full, fat cells and other cells in the GI tract initiate signals that interact with those of the central nervous system. Traditional appetite suppressants target serotonin and norepinephrine, two of the key neural transmitters in the brain. When serotonin increases, there is a greater feeling of fullness. When norepinephrine increases, appetite is decreased. Orlistate (Xenical, Alli) is the only type of weight loss pharmaceutical that works directly on the digestive tract that prevents the intestines from absorbing approximately 1/3 of fat consumed.

The most commonly prescribed amphetamine-like weight loss prescription written is for is a combination of phentermine and topiramate, sold under the brand name Qsymia. Other common isolated amphetamine-like weight loss prescription drugs include: phentermine is only prescribed for up to 12 weeks, sibutramine up to 12 months, phendimetrazine and diethylpropion. Common negative side effects of these types of weight loss drugs, however, are very similar to those of amphetamine use in general, including but not limited to: drug dependence and abuse, irritability, personality changes, insomnia, even psychosis similar to schizophrenia, dizziness, insomnia, dry mouth, and constipation.

Sudden withdrawal of many weight loss pharmaceuticals may result in severe depression. These types of drugs are also contraindicated in those diagnosed with heart disease, high blood pressure, or thyroid problems. Other potential negative side effects, on a specific pharmaceutical basis include those for phenteramine (Adipex-P, Fastin) where there are reports of patients developing pulmonary hypertension presenting with symptoms include trouble breathing, chest pain, fainting, and edema. Leaky heart valves have also been associated with phenteramine use. Diethylpropion (Tenuate) can increased the risk of convulsions in those with epilepsy, with other patients reporting hallucinations and toxic psychosis.

Even though those individuals diagnosed with obesity are often also diagnosed with high blood pressure, sibutramine (Meridia) can actually substantially raise blood pressure and/or pulse rate in some patients. Other common negative side effects specific to sibutramine include headache, dry mouth, anorexia, constipation, insomnia, runny nose, and sore throat. Because of the potential negative side effects of sibutramine, doctors are told not to prescribe this pharmaceutical for patients with a previous history of hypertension, stroke, heart disease, or severe kidney or liver disease.

In particular, orlistat (Xenical, Alli) has it's own list of specific side effects or other issues that are different from the other weight loss prescription drugs identified here. For example, when patients taking orlistat consume high-fat diets or meals negative side effects from the pharmaceutical are increased, including diarrhea, oily stools, gas, flatulence, and a decrease in the absorption of fat-soluble vitamin (A, D, E., and K). In fact, patients taking orlistat are specifically told they not should take a multivitamin containing fat-soluble vitamins with two hours' separation from the orlistat dose.

What is so important about fat soluble vitamins you might ask. Vitamin A, or retinol, supports your reproductive, digestive, urinary and immune systems, and is essential to the health of your bones, skin and eyes. Vitamin D helps your body build and maintain strong bones and teeth, and supports the effective and healthy functioning of nerves and muscles. Vitamin E protects your body organs and tissues from the damaging effects of reactive chemicals called free radicals, and the damage to the body from other chemical toxins. And finally, vitamin K is used by the body for the maintenance of bone health and integrity and is required for the liver to manufacture proteins called coagulation factors, which help your blood clot if you sustain an injury.

In addition to the nutrient deficiencies discussed throughout this chapter, weight loss pharmaceuticals carry with them a series of additional risks based on interactions with other mediations, many of which are typically used by those with weight problems as these are the individuals most likely to be diagnosed with diabetes, cardiovascular disease, and emotional issues as I've discussed throughout this section. For example, Phentermine may decrease the effectiveness of guanethidine. Tenuate may interact with blood pressure medications, insulin, and other medications such as Thorazine. Sibutramine should not be used with, or within two weeks of, monoamine oxidase inhibitors (MAOIs). Doing so may precipitate a serious and sometimes fatal side effect known as the "serotonin syndrome." Sibutramine can interact with other antidepressants, narcotic pain medication, antibiotics, and migraine medications.

Emotional health. I strongly advocate the use of various pharmaceutical agents for clients in *urgent* need of antidepressant or anti-anxiety, or other emotionally related challenges, again stressing when facing an urgent situation in order to help the person over their crisis. However, this area is typically one of the most overprescribed yet under-prescribed pharmacological areas in medicine. What I mean by this dichotomy is that antidepressants, for example, are the most common drugs prescribed. On the other hand, unless the patient states they are depressed, it is also one of the most under-prescribed areas as most doctors do not inquire the mental health status of patients with other disorders, and even more remotely among those who are in their senior years. That said, as with other risk areas, each of the pharmaceutical agents prescribed for emotional health carry their own risks, including but not limited to addiction.

Antidepressants

As is the case for most of the other health risks related to the onset of dementia that we've discussed so far, anti-depressants are also categorized into groups based upon the mode of action. In the case of antidepressants, there are five different categories of pharmaceuticals: Selective serotonin reuptake inhibitors (SSRIs), Serotonin-norepinephrine reuptake inhibitors (SNRIs), Tricyclic antidepressants (TCAs), Monoamine oxidase inhibitors (MAOIs), and Atypical agents.

Selective serotonin reuptake inhibitors (SSRIs) are the most commonly prescribed type/category of antidepressants, and are believed to reduce symptoms of depression by blocking the reabsorption (reuptake) of serotonin in the brain. Commonly prescribed selective serotonin reuptake inhibitors (SSRIs), many of which you may have heard of in television commercials or seen in advertisements in magazines include citalopram (Celexa), escitalopram (Lexapro), fluoxetine (Prozac), fluvoxamine (Luvox), fluvoxamine CR (Luvox CR), paroxetine (Paxil), paroxetine CR (Paxil CR), sertraline (Zoloft). Common negative side effects of SSRIs are known to include nausea, vomiting, diarrhea, sexual dysfunction, headache, weight gain, anxiety, dizziness, dry mouth, and trouble sleeping. Further, it has been reported that the use of SSRIs with certain over the counter pain relievers such as aspirin, ibuprofen like Motrin or Advil, naproxen such as Naprosyn, or Aleve, and prescription blood thinners such as warfarin [Coumadin]) may increase the risk of bleeding. Additionally, a condition known as serotonin syndrome can occur, which includes anxiety, restlessness, sweating, muscle spasms, shaking, fever, rapid heartbeat, vomiting, and diarrhea. Finally, there are significant risks of suicidal thoughts and actions in patients taking these pharmaceuticals.

Serotonin norepinephrine reuptake inhibitors (SNRIs) are another category of antidepressants, and they work by not only blocking the reabsorption (reuptake) of serotonin, like the SSRIs discussed above, but they also block the reabsorption (reuptake) of another neural transmitter called norepinephrine in the brain. Common SNRIs which you may have seen in television commercials or in magazine advertisements that you might recognize by their name include desvenlafaxine (Pristiq), duloxetine (Cymbalta), venlafaxine (Effexor), venlafaxine XR which is an extended release Effexor, milnacipran (Savella), and levomilnacipran (Fetzima). Negative side effects commonly reported with SNRIs include: nausea, dizziness, sexual dysfunction, tiredness and fatigue, constipation, insomnia and other sleep disturbances, anxiety, headaches, loss of appetite, abnormal bleeding, and sweating. Finally, as is the case for SSRIs, SNRIs also carry the risk of suicidal thoughts or actions in patients taking these pharmaceuticals.

Although not as commonly prescribed anymore compared to SSRIs or SNRIs, tricyclic antidepressants (TCAs) were one of the first category of antidepressants approved by the FDA. However, their mode of action is like the SNRI in that it blocks the reabsorption (reuptake) of serotonin and norepinephrine; however, TCA's also block muscarinic M1, histamine H1, and alpha-adrenergic receptors. Common tricyclic antidepressants (TCAs) that you might recognize from television commercials or in talking to people you know include amitriptyline (Elavil) which is still commonly prescribed, desipramine (Norpramin), doxepine (Sinequan), Imipramine (Tofranil), nortriptyline (Pamelor), amoxapine, clomipramine (Anafranil), maprotiline (Ludiomil), trimipramine (Surmontil), and protriptyline (Vivactil). Common negative side effects include: dry mouth, blurred vision, urinary retention, constipation, dizziness, memory impairment, delirium, tachycardia (rapid heart beat) or other heartbeat irregularities, weight gain, seizures, bone fractures, sexual dysfunction, and increased sweating. Additionally, when doctors may change medications from one category to another, it is important that TCAs are not used within 14 days of taking an MAOI antidepressant (the category discussed next).

Finally, TCAs have their own known nutrient deficiencies. For example, Coenzyme Q10 is a major known nutrient deficiency associated with TCAs, and can cause congestive heart failure, increased blood pressure, cardiomyopathy, muscle cramps, and periodontal disease. One of the reasons for these issues due to the nutrient deficiency is that CoQ10 is pivotal in the production of energy within the mitochondria of each and every cell in your body. It is involved in the production of adenosine triphosphate (ATP), which is a high energy fuel in every living cell. It is also and important antioxidant. Because it is fat-soluble, it is able to reside in the mitochondrial cell membrane where it provides protection against free radical damage to DNA. The other major nutrient deficiency associated with TCAs is vitamin B2, which will affect the mucous membranes and skin, causing a condition known as Cheilosis (cracks in the corners of the mouth). It is also common that Vitamin B2 deficiencies are found in cases where patients present with symptoms of redness, tearing, burning, and itching of the eyes, eyes that tire easily, and eyes the are very sensitive to light.

The next major category of antidepressant pharmaceuticals is referred to as monoamine oxidase inhibitors (MAOIs), which are designed to block the activity of monoamine oxidase, which is an enzyme that breaks down norepinephrine, serotonin, and dopamine in the brain and in other parts of the body. Because MAOIs have many drug and food interactions and are known to cause significant side effects compare to SSRIs or SNRIs, they are not as widely prescribed anymore. Three of the more common MAOIs are: phenelzine (Nardil), selegiline (Emsam), and tranylcypromine (Parnate). Some of the more common side effects include significant reductions in blood pressure, dizziness upon standing, fatigue, weight gain, and sexual side effects. Additionally, as with the case of other antidepressant pharmaceuticals in other categories, there is a strong risk of suicidal thoughts, ideations, or actions with the use of MAOIs. With MAOIs, however, there are specific dietary precautions that patients must be aware of or they could lead to a hypertensive crisis. Specifically, patients taking MAOIs with foods or beverages that contain tyramine could raise their blood pressure to dangerous levels. Common foods that contain tyramine include: wine, aged cheese, sauerkraut, cured meats, draft beer, and soy products to name a few.

The last category we'll discuss are known as Atypical antidepressants. This category is a type of "catch-all" category for antidepressants that don't fit into any of the other established pharmacological categories, and each one of the pharmaceuticals in this category have their own mechanism of action as well while they affect the levels of serotonin, norepinephrine and dopamine within the brain. However, like other antidepressants, atypical antidepressants affect the levels of dopamine, serotonin, and norepinephrine in the brain. Some of the more common atypical antidepressants include Brintellix and Viibryd, which are like SSRIs by inhibiting the reuptake of serotonin, but they also act on serotonin receptors as well. Other atypical antidepressants also include bupropion (Wellbutrin) which is also an anti-convulsant and can be used to reduce hot-flashes in menopausal women, mirtazapine (Remeron), nefazodone (Serzone), and trazodone (Desyrel, Oleptro), which is also used as a sleep aide. Given medications in this class have unique properties, their side effect profile also varies. Some common side effects include dry mouth, constipation, dizziness, and lightheadedness. However, medication specific effects include those experienced when taking mirtazapine and trazodone cause drowsiness and are usually taken at bedtime (which is why the later is often prescribed for sleep), mirtazapine and trazodone may cause abnormal heart rhythms which can be life threatening, trazodone can also cause priapism in men (painful and prolonged erection), nefazodone may cause life-threatening liver failure, and bupropion should not be used in patients with known seizure disorders (despite the fact it is an anti-convulsant), eating disorders, and within 2 weeks of using MAOIs. Finally, as has been the case with antidepressants in all other categories, there is a significant risk of suicidal thoughts, ideations, and actions when taking an atypical antidepressant.

Anti-anxiety drugs

There are upwards of 80 different prescription anti-anxiety pharmaceuticals on the market today. Not surprisingly, anti-anxiety pharmaceuticals are also categorized into different groups based on mechanism of action. The three most commonly prescribed types of anxiety medication are antidepressants, anti-anxiety medications (also known as anxiolytics), and beta-blockers. Antidepressants and anxiolytic medications work primarily by affecting the balance of certain chemicals in the brain known as neurotransmitters. Beta-blockers and other types of drugs are used to address the physical symptoms that may accompany an anxiety attack. It is also interesting to note that many first-generation antihistamines are also used to help relieve symptoms associated with anxiety simply due to their sedative effects. Remember, the key to the use of and understanding anti-anxiety medications is that they do not cure anxiety disorders, they simply modify the various chemicals and neurotransmitters in the brain to help control the symptoms associated with anxiety.

One of the major pharmaceutical groupings that most are familiar with within the anxiolytic category of anti-anxiety medications are benzodiazepines. This is a term you may have heard on television medical shows, or seen in commercials. The term benzodiazepine is essentially synonymous with the term tranquilizers, and these are the most widely prescribed type of medication for anxiety. One of the reasons for their widespread use is their rapid mechanism of action, with patients typically responding in a calmer state within 30 minutes from ingesting the pharmaceutical. Some of the most common benzodiazepines prescribed include: alprazolam (Xanax), chlordiazepoxide (Librium), clonazepam (Klonopin), diazepam (Valium), and lorazepam (Ativan). Although they are widely prescribed, these pharmaceuticals come with a huge cautionary note: Benzodiazepines are highly physically additive and should only be used for short-term relief. Some of the other common side effects of benzodiazepines include: drowsiness, dizziness, poor balance or coordination, slurred speech, trouble concentrating, memory problems, confusion and difficulty with cognitive thinking, stomach upset, nausea and other digestive issues, headache, and blurred vision. Of special note are the side effects experienced by children, the elderly, and people with developmental disabilities when prescribed benzodiazepines, which mirror those associated with anxiety in the first place. These include: increased anxiety, irritability, agitation, aggression, rage, mania, impulsive behavior, and hallucinations.

Of particular concern, particularly based on our subject matter of preventing dementia, when benzodiazepines are given to older individuals. As highlighted in the previous paragraph, even small doses can cause confusion, amnesia, loss of balance, and cognitive impairment that actually looks like dementia. *Additionally, long-term benzodiazepine use also increases the risk of Alzheimer's disease and dementia.*

SSRIs used to treat depression are also often used to treat anxiety as well, including those pharmaceuticals discussed in our earlier section on SSRIs above. The most commonly prescribed SSRIs for anxiety are: Prozac, Zoloft, Paxil, Lexapro, and Celexa. They carry the same negative side effects when prescribed for anxiety as they do when they are prescribed for depression.

Buspirone (BuSpar), is a newer anti-anxiety drug that acts as a mild tranquilizer. However, whereas benzodiazepines are popular because they are fast acting, buspirone is slow acting, and actually takes approximately two weeks before patients can see that the pharmaceutical is actually working for them. However, whereas most benzodiazepines are sedating, buspirone is only mildly sedating and better tolerated by most individuals and only carries minimal withdrawal side effects. However, buspirone actually has a greater number of common side effects than benzodiazepines, including nausea and vomiting, headaches, dizziness, drowsiness, weight gain, upset stomach, constipation or diarrhea, nervousness and increased anxiety, and dry mouth.

The pharmaceutical remedies for the risks associated with the onset of dementia discussed in this chapter including numbers of types of drugs available when mentioned, are representative of those pharmaceuticals available and approved by the FDA for use in the US. This does not include those pharmaceuticals manufactured and approved for use in other countries, such as Great Britain, Canada, China, India, and so forth. In each of these countries there are many other pharmaceuticals available, and pharmaceutical manufacturing plants in business. If you do the math, you can see there are thousands upon thousands of pharmaceutical agents available worldwide to combat risks associated with the onset of dementia.

I've not mentioned all of the nutrient depletions associated with all of the medications specified in this chapter, but it is critical to highlight that each of these medications carry additional significant and similar nutrient depletions and carry other problems as well. For example, often dihydropyridines, as well as other pharmaceuticals mentioned throughout this section, grapefruit juice has been noted as causing a problem. Here's what happens, grapefruit juice will increase the effects of many medications according to a pharmakinetic measure referred to as the area under the curve (AUC). Every pharmaceutical has its own unique set of specific subtleties and side effects. Most doctors and/or pharmacists might mention a few of the possible side effects, or you'll see them in patient information handouts that come with your medication, but the list you will be provided is far from complete.

It is also critical to remember that you are a wonderfully unique individual. The side effects that affect 50 out of 100 patients in a clinical study may or may not be what you are experiencing. In fact, you may have a side effect that has not been reported by the pharmaceutical company and more likely than not, in this situation both the doctor and pharmacist will tell you what you are experiencing has nothing to do with the medication when it does.

And, if they do acknowledge there is an issue with the pharmaceutical agent, here's what will most likely happen nine times out of: most doctors will change you to another prescription in the same family of pharmaceuticals, meaning that nine times out of ten the new medication will be in the same family of drugs so you will still be likely to experience a series of similar negative side effects due to the chemical structure of the new drug and mechanism of action.

Here is another important issue: if you are seeing several doctors for various health challenges, it is likely that you will also be on multiple pharmaceuticals; or they may all even be prescribed by one doctor. Your pharmacist should have a digital profile created for you showing all medications you are taking, and potential interaction alerts should come up the minute the pharmacy technician enters the prescription you just set out to fill. But of course this is limited to what that specific pharmacy is filling for you. If you get one prescription filled from CVS, but another from Walgreens, each of their lists will be incomplete. Therefore, in addition to negative side effects of a single medication, potential drug interaction warnings are critical - the wrong combination can kill you. They can work with each other, or they can work against each other, or they may even combine to create a lethal combination. It is up to you to do your own research. The website www.drugs.com is an excellent place to start.

Further, it is critical to remember that pharmaceutical medications make widespread changes throughout your body when mitigating a specific health issue, such as high blood pressure or high cholesterol, in addition to lowering your blood pressure or cholesterol level. These could represent sub-clinical negative side effects, or negative side effects that cannot readily be identified. Some you may feel, some you many not even feel but they are there. But either way, there are a myriad of effects that take place throughout your body just from taking one little pill, and those changes are not always healthful. In many ways it's like trying to fix one problem and causing another. For example, many individuals with autoimmune disorders such as lupus, require the long-term use of corticosteroids. This leads to osteoporosis and bone degeneration. Many individuals I know who have been on prednisone, for example, have had to undergo numerous hip or knee joint replacements.

I also believe it is critical that you are an informed consumer. The more you research, the more you are in a position to question and discuss medications that are prescribed from a position of knowing and advocating for yourself. Why is your doctor prescribing that medication for you rather than another one? When can you expect a significant improvement, and how can you tell if it is working? What are the potential risks? What are the interactions? How long will you need to take this medication? And I implore you – the answer to these questions is not "We'll have to wait and see how you respond."

I started this chapter by stating that although I am a naturopath, I believe there is a time and place for pharmaceutical use. However, based on just the limited writing here in this chapter related to specific risk areas related to dementia and Alzheimer's disease, it is the side effects and potentially secondary risks related to use of the pharmaceuticals that you, and you alone, have to assess. Is the cure worse than the problem? Is it changing one risk for another? Are there any other methods that can be used to correct the primary risk related to dementia and Alzheimer's disease such as high blood pressure, that can be addressed through mitigation actions that do not include pharmaceutical use? These are all questions and issues you should address either with your doctor or in the privacy of your own home as you take responsibility for your own healthcare.

My personal approach to my own healthcare is to address a disease or disorder by employing natural mitigation strategies, including diet and supplementation. I'd rather do all I can to work WITH my body in the most healthful, safe, and effective manner possible first to correct a situation, presuming it is not an emergency situation. Only if after all attempts at a natural solution fail, then the most conservative pharmaceutical approach should be identified and discussed.

Chapter Six: Safe, healthy, and effective natural alternatives

Just as we reviewed the varied pharmaceutical medications a doctor is most likely to recommend for the risks associated with dementia, this chapter will take the same approach, but review natural alternatives to actual pharmaceuticals that alleviate or mitigate these risks.

Before this chapter highlights the major natural treatment remedies associated with those risks related to the onset of dementia, as compared to the pharmaceuticals detailed in the previous chapter, I also want to note the following: I prefer working with single remedies rather than a complex made up of different herbs. Most of the reason there are so many bottles on the shelves of health food stores is because companies put together so many different complexes where ingredients may sound like they belong together, but in reality, all the ingredients may or may not work together synergistically. I am very fond of homeopathic remedies as well as herbs and other supplements such as amino acids and other similar compounds the body naturally produces, however, this chapter is designed to give you an idea of the types of natural treatments available. None of the sections will provide an exhaustive list. Given that virtually all natural remedies have side effects and their own subtle nuances of how they work, what they work best with, what they should not be used with, and so forth, I rarely recommend products that group ingredients into one capsule, tablet, or tincture. As a result, the presentation on natural remedies in this chapter will focus strictly on individual remedies, rather than a specific product name that incorporates a complex of ingredients in their own recipe.

Exposure to heavy metals. This is an area where natural medicine seriously excels in my opinion over traditional medicine. However, that said, I believe that traditional medicine considers toxic levels of heavy metals as being far higher than one would from a natural health perspective. Remember from our discussion on risks in Chapter Three; the minimal levels of risk from amalgam fillings, for example, are enough to cause serious neurological damage. That said, what are some of the natural alternatives to pharmaceutical chelation agents.

One of the most well known natural source to remove heavy metals, is chlorella. You can readily find standard chlorella capsules or pressed pills, even powder on the shelves of most health food stores. Chlorella consists of 60% protein in the form of amino acids. In fact, there are 22 different amino acids, all but 8, the essential amino acids, can be produced inside our body. The 8 essential amino acids must be consumed from food. If any of these essential amino acids are lacking, the others cannot function. Chlorella contains 19 out of 22 different amino acids including all 8 of the essential amino acids (leucine, valine, lysine, phenylalanine, threonine, isoleucine, methionine, tryptophan). As a result, chlorella is considered a complete protein.

This is a perfect example of how natural remedies are more healthful than prescription remedies. Whereas prescription medications only contain an active ingredient, with the rest of the ingredients considered inactive or excipients; very rarely are there ingredients in a pharmaceutical that will support the body. As you will see in the cases of the healthier options, such as chlorella, you are getting significant health benefits in addition to mitigating the disease or disorder for which you are seeking a remedy. For example, in addition to the full protein structure and heavy metal elimination, chlorella also supports the human genetic material in each of our cells offering a huge protecting mechanism, including slowing down the aging process.

Additionally, chlorella maintains and repairs healthy cells, increases energy levels, stimulates growth of new cells, supports immune function, and stimulates the maturation and growth in children who have not yet reached their full, adult size. Finally, unlike many metal detoxification products or protocols, works on the friendly lactic bacteria in the gut by fostering it to increase/multiply at four times the usual rate, thereby improving digestion and the absorption of nutrients into the bloodstream.

This last benefit is very important. Most individuals have digestive yeast and leaking gut problems you may or many not be aware of. Firstly, if you have leaky gut syndrome, anything that passes through your digestive tract will ultimately also be transmitted, or leaked, from the gut to the blood stream and circulate throughout your body. Ideally, you need to knit the gut back together again, seal the leaks as it were, before you begin a heavy metal detoxification program. And you also have to eliminate digestive yeast and candida first. Otherwise you are creating more problems for yourself.

The reason you must proceed with your natural approach to heavy metal detoxification in the proper order of steps, as a full program, is because mercury and other heavy metals feed yeast. So, if you are working to detoxify yourself from heavy metals, and are concerned about amalgam fillings as related to the risk associated with developing dementia, it is important not to compromise your health in other areas, such as digestively, or even systemically with toxins being carried into your bloodstream and carried throughout your body. Therefore, it is critical to work with a natural healthcare professional to do more than a simple yeast cleanse, but to also support healing leaky gut syndrome BEFORE you initiate any heavy metal detoxification programs.

Especially when looking at a heavy metal detoxification protocol, it is not something you will achieve with one box of chlorella off the health food store shelf. Ideally, although significant reductions in heavy metals are achieved within the first month to two months; a full program could take between 7 and 12 months.

The product I recommend for heavy metal detoxification, and use myself, is one specifically developed for professional use that is based on a micronized chlorella to more effectively and efficiently get bind to heavy metals, and removes them through the urinary tract. The micronized chlorella is more effective because the cell walls are broken and can thus be more effective in the chelation process. The company manufacturing this product also offers a full range of support products for the liver, the digestive system, and endocrine system throughout the detoxification protocol. All ingredients for all products are 100% herbal, and nutrient rich.

As a result, instead of the traditional list of potential side effects one sees with pharmaceutical medications, the only side effect of the detox protocol I recommend (again, where there is full support of the liver, and so forth), is a very mildly increased feeling of being easily aggravated. This typically resolves within 24 hours, with no other lasting effects. When taking this product, there is relatively lengthy period of time from initiation of the program until the maximum dosage is obtained. Therefore, if any feelings of aggravation are felt, all the individual has to do is go back to the previous dosage and not continue to increase anymore.

Atherosclerosis

There are a number of natural remedies that can be found for atherosclerosis. For example, fish oil, rich in omega-3 fatty acids is known to reduce inflammation, lower blood lipids (especially triglycerides), improve blood viscosity, and normalize heart rhythms. Some reports suggest that taking these supplements can reduce cardiovascular mortality by as much as 45%. While I cannot state this is true or not, I can say fish oil is a great supplement for a number of issues and that it does help reducing inflammation and improves cardiovascular function, it will help issues related to atherosclerosis. However, it is important to look at where the fish oil is derived from. For example, if it is sourced in the Pacific, you are more likely to find more heavy metal toxins from pollution compared to Norwegian derived fish oils. The same principle also holds on whether the source is farm raised or wild caught. Farm raised fish and sea food is likely to be genetically modified; with wild caught fish there is a significantly reduced likelihood that any genetic modifications will present (pollution issues aside).

Coenzyme Q10, also commonly referred to as CoQ10, is an excellent antioxidant, which means it prevents damage by free radicals in the form of oxidation, maintains healthy blood vessels, lowers blood pressure, and has been evidenced as supporting optimal functioning of the heart muscle. However, like all supplements, CoQ10 is not for everyone. There are potential side effects; for example, mild nausea has been reported with the use of this supplement.

Garlic is also an excellent antioxidants and increases nitric oxide production, all of which is very good at reducing endothelial cell dysfunction. Endothelial cells are the cells that line the blood vessels, and all other organs. While garlic is heralded as being one of the great cure-alls, ranging from cancer to infections, one website I saw on natural health and atherosclerosis recommending garlic stated, and I quote: "In any case, garlic probably won't hurt you." Remember what I said about 20 pages of contraindications and warnings? This brings up another important point. It's very easy for us to all look to the internet and try to do our research, or we see postings on social media on best alternative or natural remedies for this or that. Accepting blanket guidance and suggestions from these sources without knowing who they're really coming from, and not consulting with a qualified natural healthcare professional can be very dangerous! Back to remedies....

Trimethylglycine (TMG) is a natural compound that lowers homocysteine levels. Not everyone is familiar with what homocysteine is. So let me give you a very quick lesson on what it is and what can happen. Homocysteine is an amino acid that, in excess amounts, is irritating to the arteries and is strongly associated with inflammation and hardening of the arteries. In fact, if you think of it this way, the effect of homocysteine is almost like sandpaper on the endothelial tissue lining your arteries. It creates mini-abrasions that are actually repaired with cholesterol deposits, much like you'd use spackle on a wall in your home. That is why the levels of homocysteine in your blood are actually a good measure of cardiovascular and atherosclerosis risk. If your homocysteine level is too high, TMG can help lower your levels, thus helping to maintain irritant free arteries and lessen the amount of cholesterol deposits formed that lead to plaque and narrowing of arteries.

Curcumin, the active ingredient in turmeric, is an herb known to possess tremendous anti-inflammatory abilities. Therefore, it should not surprise you to know that curcumin is also highly reputed as helpful to prevent buildup of plaque, therefore acting as a proactive agent to prevent the onset of atherosclerosis leading to blocked arteries, stroke or heart attack. Curcumin also has high levels of vitamin B6, which is considered an essential vitamin in maintaining optimal homocysteine levels.

While a lot of supplements in this section are often recommended for a variety of purposes, which may or may not be related, one of my favorites for circulation and heart health in general, that also works great when there are potential issues with high homocysteine levels and fears related to cholesterol deposits on endothelial tissue, is Nattokinase. Nattokinase is actually an enzyme that can break down the adhesive substance that can make arterial plaque sticky. In this way, it provides a preventative and reversing effect on blood clotting and plaque build up in the arteries. Nattokinase is a powerful proteolytic enzyme that has fibrinolytic (anti-clotting) health benefits. A similar proteolytic enzyme is Serrapeptase.

High cholesterol

There are a number of natural remedies for high cholesterol. Red Yeast Rice is just one of many. However, the key is the monacolin K compound known as *monascus purpureaus*, which is the a red-pigmented yeast grown on the actual white rice when left to ferment. In addition to natural monacolins, red yeast rice contains the phystosterols, beta-sitosterol, campesterol, and stigmasterol, which are varied plant based sterols, (also highly recommended as a natural treatment option for high cholesterol), as well as isoflavones and trace minerals, all of which can contribute to cardiovascular health. In fact, this is a perfect example of pharmaceutical drugs closely copying or replicating natural treatments. In this case, lovastatin, discussed in the previous chapter as a statin-based pharmaceutical for lowering cholesterol, possesses the same type of compound as the monacolin K found in red yeast rice.

Plant stanols and sterols (such as beta-sitosterol and sitostanol) are naturally-occurring substances found in certain plants, as highlighted above in the red yeast rice, but are available as stand alone remedies. Plant stanols and sterols are actually similar in structure to cholesterol and it is thought that are effective because they help block the absorption of cholesterol from the intestines, significantly reduced total cholesterol and LDL cholesterol.

Artichoke leaf extract, often referred to simply as ALE has been reported to help raise your "good" cholesterol and lower "bad" cholesterol. Once again, food based, artichokes also contain a compound called cynarine, believed to increase bile production in the liver and speed the flow of bile from the gallbladder, both of which may increase the elimination of cholesterol from the body with no reported adverse effects.

Policosinol, and guggulipid are also natural treatment remedies known to reduce cholesterol. In fact, guggulipid, the gum resin of the mukul myrrh tree, has been shown to significantly reduce blood levels of both total cholesterol and LDL cholesterol.

Niacin is also known as vitamin B-3, and is known to help raise your good (HDL) cholesterol levels by a third, and also lower triglycerides, another fat that increases heart disease risk. Niacin also lowers a substance called lipoprotein A, a fatty protein that is known as a risk factor for atherosclerosis. Niacin supplements can make your skin flushed and prickly feeling, and might cause nausea.

Personally, I like to see my clients consume as many natural treatment remedies directly from their food-based form. For example, many supplement manufacture their supplements only from food-based ingredients. Simply put, the body knows what to do with food, that's how we were designed. Our bodies don't know what to do with something manufactured in a laboratory. In the case of niacin, foods that are naturally very high in niacin include liver, chicken, tuna, and salmon.

For this section as well as throughout this eBook, any mention of foods high in a specific nutrient or natural remedy are listed here without regard to alignment with any specific diet or potential health restriction you might have. This is another reason to consult your qualified natural health practitioner before not only using any supplement, but also before beginning treatment with a specific food source for therapeutic purposes.

Although I've highlighted the risks of taking natural remedies without consulting a qualified natural health professional when we've talked about garlic, niacin also presents another good example. There are significant contraindications for the use of niacin, as it can increase the effect of high blood pressure medication (thus causing low blood pressure, dizziness, and possible fainting), or cause nausea, indigestion, gas, diarrhea, cause or trigger gout, and worsen peptic ulcers, liver inflammation, and high blood sugar. However, the most frequently noted negative side effect is skin flushing or hot flashes, which is caused by widening of blood vessels. Most people only notice this when they initially start taking niacin, and can be reduced if the niacin is taken with meals, rather than on an empty stomach. The flushing will naturally discontinue to be a problem within several days of maintaining your normal niacin-based treatment schedule.

Another option to food-based supplements is to ingest the specific foods that are helpful for a problem itself. For example, soluble fiber appears to reduce LDL cholesterol by reducing cholesterol absorption in the intestines, basically binding with cholesterol so that it is excreted as solid waste. Although you can get soluble fiber in supplement form, such as psyllium powder, I prefer clients seeking to increase their soluble fiber intake do it from food sources. For example, many foods considered high in soluble fiber include: oats, barley, rye, peas, flaxseed, beans, and some fruits such as apples, prunes, and berries, as well as some vegetables, including carrots, brussel sprouts, broccoli, and yams. I fact, just 5 – 10 grams a day of soluble fiber has been found to decrease LDL cholesterol by approximately 5%.

High blood pressure
Several supplements are excellent for helping to reduce high blood pressure. For example, magnesium. Magnesium works to relax smooth muscle tissues that can then more readily dilate the arteries and reduce blood pressure. What is particularly interesting, in addition to zinc deficiencies, many blood pressure medications cause magnesium deficiencies, thus working to actually increase high blood pressure in the process, fighting against the prescription you've been given.

Hibiscus is another natural remedy that is used lower blood pressure. The way it works is interesting and you can see parallels to pharmaceuticals discussed in the last chapter. First, hibiscus acts as a diuretic, which draws sodium from the bloodstream, thus decreasing the pressure on the arterial walls. Even more interesting is how it can mimic angiotensin converting enzyme (ACE) inhibitors.. As a result of this inhibition, blood vessels relax and blood volume is lowered, decreasing blood pressure. While certainly not as potent as those ACE drugs prescribed, it can still be surprisingly effective.

Hawthorn is another herb used to lower blood pressure, and is also used in many remedies targeting the cardiovascular system, including those for lowering cholesterol. The major compounds inherent in hawthorn gives it most of its value is called flavonoids, namely, oligomeric procyandins (OPC's) and quercetin. Flavonoids are known for possessing a great many benefits to systems throughout the body, however, the ones most researched are those pertaining to the cardiovascular system and heart health reducing or eliminating arrhythmias and palpitations, can improve the function of capillaries, and regulate glucose metabolism. For purposes of our discussion, hawthorn is great for reducing arterial blood pressure and the risk of hypertension by widening of the blood vessels, which ultimately reduces the pressure of the blood.

Diabetes
As has been mentioned at the beginning of this chapter, and I believe you are sensing at this point: there are a number of different natural remedies available for the treatment of just about anything. As germane to our discussion of risks associated with the onset of dementia, type 2 diabetes is a major one, as it is also associated as a causal or related risk to all the other risks ranging from high cholesterol, atherosclerosis, high blood pressure, and obesity.

One of the remedies available for the treatment of type 2 diabetes is chromium which metabolizes carbohydrates. Chromium is actually an essential mineral required to produce something called glucose tolerance factor, which is a compound in our bodies that improves how we use insulin. However, there is always the caution that too much chromium can have the inverse effect, and like some pharmaceuticals designed to treat type 2 diabetes, actually leave the person in a hypoglycemic state, where the person's blood sugar is too low rather than too high.

Vanadium is another naturally occurring mineral compound produced in humans. Vanadium helps to balance blood sugar levels in cases with type 1 and type 2 diabetes, increasing their own sensitivity to insulin causing it to work more efficiently, and thus lowers the individuals' actual need for insulin.

Cinnamon is an excellent natural remedy for type 2 diabetes for many individuals. Essentially, cinnamon extracts can improve sugar metabolism, triggering insulin release, which also boosts cholesterol metabolism. In fact, cinnamon has been linked to lowering blood sugar levels in Chinese medicine for hundreds of years.

In the chapter on risks associated with a greater likelihood of developing dementia we briefly referred to anxiety and depression, and the last chapter reviewed the most common US pharmaceuticals used to treat them. This section will briefly cover natural treatment options for these two common challenges.

Anxiety

The most common types of herbs for anxiety include kava kava, passion flower, chamomile, lemon balm, and valerian root. Specifically, kava kava, often referred to as just kava, is considered one of the major natural treatment options for working with anxiety. The primary ingredient in kava, kavalactone, reportedly improves GABA levels and as a result, prevents epinephrine from overwhelming the body while leaving serotonin and other important neurotransmitters untouched. Although kava has no addictive properties, there are a number of warnings and contraindications. For example, when taken in high doses or in combination with other herbs, kava can promote extreme drowsiness, and like many anti-anxiety pharmaceuticals should not be mixed with alcohol.

Passionflower is similar to kava, but is not as strong as kava is known to be. Passionflower also affects GABA production and regulation, thus producing anti-anxiety effects. Passionflower may not be strong enough, however, for those who deal with anxiety on a regular daily basis. Again, all the more need to consult with a qualified natural health professional before starting on any natural treatment protocol

Most people associate chamomile with a pleasant light herbal tea. However, chamomile has similar antianxiety properties as many pharmaceuticals designed to treat anxiety. For example, one of the compounds in chamomile, known as *matricaria recutita*, actually bind to the same receptors within the brain as valium does, thus making chamomile a good natural treatment option with fewer side effects than kava.

Lemon balm, also known as the herb Melissa, is one of my favorite herbs, mostly because of its anti-inflammatory and anti-viral properties. However, lemon balm is also known to reduce stress and anxiety. There is a general caution in using lemon balm for anxiety. However, while we in Western society typically believe when we don't see or feel results from a medication (pharmaceutical or natural) that we need to take more, this can be dangerous with lemon balm. Too much lemon balm can actually increase levels of anxiety.

Valerian root and magnesium do not actually fall into the category of natural anti-anxiety remedies like kava or passionflower, but both can be used to reduce muscle tension and agitation which often accompany and/or present as symptoms associated with anxiety. If symptoms of restlessness and agitation are reduced often the generalized feeling of being anxious will also dissipate. However, a word of caution about valerian root. Valerian root can promote depression in many people and should not be used independently without the supervision of a qualified natural health professional. Similarly, too much magnesium can lead to digestive issues including nausea and diarrhea.

Depression

There are a number of vitamins and supplements for depression, which is why in many of the supplements under a brand name that have multiple ingredients, you'll generally see vitamins as well. For example, you're more than likely to see B vitamins, including folic acid, vitamin B12, and vitamin B6, as well as, traditional herbs, such as St. John's wort. Vitamin B12 is known to play an important role in the production of neural transmitters affecting anxiety and depression, including serotonin, dopamine, and epinephrine.

St. John's wort is typically one of the first herbal remedies individuals with depression turn to who seek a natural alternative to their prescription antidepressant. Research has shown St. John's wort to be as effective in some studies as Prozac, however, it typically takes approximately two months before relief is achieved. St. John's wort should be used with caution; some individuals find St. John's wort actually increases their depression, causes or increases anxiety, panic attacks, dizziness, nausea, and spikes in blood pressure. Additional cautions about the use of St. John's wort report it should not be taken with anti-retroviral medications, or other antidepressant medications, especially SSRIs like Prozac or Celexa. Finally, believe it or not, St. John's wort reduces the effectiveness of birth control pills.

L-Tryptophan is an amino acid that is the precursor to 5-HTP which then converts to serotonin. As such, L-Tryptophan has been found to be as effective for depression as antidepressant drugs and is also good for treating a wide variety of mental health conditions including anxiety, ADHD, seasonal affective disorder, eating disorders, and memory loss. L-Tryptophan is found in high-protein foods like meat, poultry, fish, and eggs. Although I prefer clients get their supplements and nutrients from food sources, the exception to the rule is L-Tryptophan. Believe it or not, L-tryptophan in supplement form typically works better than when ingested from food. Paradoxically, protein blocks serotonin synthesis and, surprisingly, both tryptophan and serotonin levels drop after eating a meal containing protein, which are typically the very foods were high levels of L-Tryptophan are found. While the tryptophan in food is completely safe, L-Tryptophan supplements should not be taken along with SSRIs.

5-HTP works to help provide the body more of the raw materials it needs to make more serotonin. 5-HTP is best used with someone who has both depression and anxiety. While 5-HTP may sound like a wonderful option to pharmaceutical antidepressants, there are cautions and warning associated with this as well. Specifically, 5-HTP should never be taken with other antidepressants, sleeping pills, anti-anxiety medications, or mixed with numerous natural remedies including kava, valerian, L-tryptophan, SAM-e, or St. John's wort, which can lead to serotonin syndrome. And lastly, 5-HTP is not advised for long-term use since, while it increases serotonin, it decreases dopamine levels. Low dopamine is an often overlooked cause of depression that is also linked to addictions of all kinds. While you can find food sources for L-Tryptophan, 5-HTP can only be consumed from a dietary supplement.

SAMe stands for S-adenosylmethionine, and is a naturally occurring chemical in the body based on the amino acid methionine which, like many of the supplements presented here, help enhance or support a number of neurotransmitters. Unlike a number of other supplements discussed here such as St. Johns wort which takes approximately two months to work, SAMe works much quicker, often lifting a depressed mood within days rather than weeks. Although SAM-e can boost the effectiveness of SSRIs, you should not mix prescription antidepressants or antianxiety medications, or with drugs that affect serotonin release such as levodopa, Demerol, or Ultram, or the over-the-counter cough remedy Robitussin DM. When SAM-e is taken with any of these drugs, the potential exists for serotonin levels to get too high, which can lead to a rare but potentially fatal condition known as serotonin syndrome.

Acetyl-l-carnitine is a synthesized form of the amino acid l-carnitine, and is a natural antidepressant that brings depression relief fast by increasing acetylcholine, the primary neurotransmitter of memory and learning, to improve mental clarity, focus, and memory.

Finally, rhodiola rosea is another herb often used as a natural antidepressant. It's particularly useful for depression caused by seasonal affective disorder. Like SAM-e, rhodiola rosea reduces depression symptoms faster than pharmaceutical antidepressants and some other natural supplements, such as St. John's wort, often providing relief within one week.

Before I get into discussions on a health lifestyle and diet, since we're still talking about natural treatments as an alternative to pharmaceuticals, I'd like to discuss healthful remedies for smoking cessation, and obesity.

Smoking cessation

Gamma-Aminobutyric acid (γ-Aminobutyric acid), more commonly referred to simply as GABA is the chief inhibitory neurotransmitter in the mammalian central nervous system. It plays the principal role in reducing neuronal excitability throughout the nervous system. Since GABA plays a role in inhibiting dopamine production, some research suggests GABA may help target nicotine dependency by reducing the pleasure derived from smoking a cigarette while simultaneously promoting a sense of focus and calm in the individual. The combination of these two is believed to help promote smoking cessation efforts. Nicotine, the key stimulant in cigarettes that leads to addiction, is a stimulant. It causes the neurons to start firing at an abnormally high rate. GABA seems to help normalize activity in your brain by slowing it down from the nicotine high.

While L-Tryptophan may not promote smoking cessation directly, it is a supplement that can help mitigate or reduce some of the symptoms associated with quitting smoking. For example, individuals who take L-Tryptophan report that it promotes relaxation, helps them maintain a positive mood and get a good night's sleep, and is known to reduce cravings for carbohydrates which is a common side effect when one quits smoking cigarettes.

5-HTP increases the production of the neurotransmitter serotonin. In cases related to smoking cigarettes, research has reported that serotonin is yet another neurotransmitter that increases with nicotine use. Some symptoms of nicotine withdrawal may stem from the fact that you have less serotonin in your system than you're used to, which could be what leads to mood issues such as depression. Therefore, 5-HTP is often a healthful supplement to reduce symptoms associated with nicotine withdrawal.

Weight loss

Weight loss is one of the most effective lifestyle changes for controlling a number of the risks we're discussing in this book. For example, mitigating high blood pressure through weight loss demonstrates that losing just 10 can help reduce your blood pressure. It's no wonder that there are so many natural products targeting weight loss!

A number of supplements provide natural weight loss support, and like their pharmaceutical counterparts, work to suppress appetite or fat absorption in different ways. For example, chitosan is actually a sugar derived from the hard outer layers of lobsters, crabs, and shrimp that is reported to block fats and cholesterol from getting absorbed by your body. As with the case of many diet aides, potential negative side effects include digestive issues and constipation. However, in addition to potential negative side effects, chitosan must not be used by individuals who are allergic to shellfish as it will cause a serious and possibly life threatening reaction.

Chromium picolinate is a wonderful all around diet aid, in that it enhances insulin, a hormone that's important for turning food into energy. Chromium picolinate is reported to suppress the appetite, increase metabolism to burn more calories, reduce body fat, and increase lean muscle mass.

Conjugated Linoleic Acid (CLA) is also another wonderful diet aide, that curbs body fat and reduces hunger. While this is a wonderful supplement, there are some reports that long-term use by those who are obese can increase insulin resistance, which can lead to or exacerbate type 2 diabetes, and potentially increase cholesterol.

Hoodia is from a plant grown in an African dessert, and is a wonderful appetite suppressant with few reported negative side effects.

Glucomannan, derived from the konjac plant, is a dietary source of fiber that works to help an individual lose weight by acting as a fat blocker, preventing the absorption of fat. It is important to note that because glucomannan is a fiber, it can reduce the ability of the body to absorb other medications, particularly if they are fat-based.

Many trendy supplements on the market have recently claimed that green tea extract is the greatest weight loss aide available. Supposedly it curbs the appetite while simultaneously raising the metabolism to burn more fat. Given it also has excitatory properties, (as do most that will raise your metabolism), this is a product I rarely recommend. In fact, negative side effects include: agitation, insomnia, dizziness, gas, bloating, vomiting, and diarrhea. Green coffee extract falls into the same category, with side effects including headaches, nervousness, abnormal heart rhythms, and insomnia. You may notice a trend here. Although these are included here as natural treatment options for the risk of obesity associated with the development of dementia, I strongly urge you to be cautious using either of these products and before doing so, that you consult your professional natural health practitioner.

Proactive healthcare

With a combination of healthful alternatives to prescription medication, incorporating a healthy lifestyle into your daily healthcare plan can significantly reduce the risks and/or impact of the risks associated with developing dementia.

Exercise

We live in a very sedentary society; we're sitting eating and then using our electronic devices, especially children. However, incorporating a regular physical activity program of at least 30 minutes most days of the week has been shown to lower your blood pressure by 4 to 9 millimeters of mercury (mm Hg). It's important to be consistent because if you stop exercising, your blood pressure can rise again. If you have slightly high blood pressure (prehypertension), exercise can help you avoid developing full-blown hypertension. If you already have hypertension, regular physical activity can bring your blood pressure down to safer levels. The best types of exercise for lowering blood pressure include walking, jogging, cycling, swimming or dancing. Strength training also can help reduce blood pressure.

Exercise is also known to lower cholesterol levels. For example, the American Heart Association suggests at least 150 minutes of moderate exercise, or 75 minutes of vigorous exercise, per week. You can mix up moderate and vigorous activity if you'd like. Some individuals need a low impact program; others can handle a more rigorous high-impact approach.

Most people can readily tolerate those exercises considered moderate level, including walking briskly (3 miles per hour or faster), bicycling (10 miles per hour or slower), playing tennis (doubles), or even gardening. As you can see, walking or gardening, should be readily achievable sources of exercise, whereas bicycle riding or tennis are a bit more active.

One key to walking is to listen to upbeat music while you are walking; you will more than likely increase your pace to an appropriate rate of 3 miles per hour or faster as your body works to move consistent with the beat of the music.

For those who can tolerate a vigorous activity program, appropriate exercise programs might include: Examples of vigorous-intensity exercise include: race walking (also known as speed walking), jogging, or running, swimming laps, playing tennis (singles), aerobic dancing, bicycling (10 miles per hour or faster), or hiking uphill.

However, before initiating any exercise program, it is critical to consult with your physician or natural health practitioner, explain your goals to them, and ask them to suggest the appropriate level of activity to start out with, and together develop a plan for increasing duration and intensity. This is particularly important if you are suffering from any cardiovascular issues.

Diet

For all of the health risks associated with the onset of dementia that we've discussed, initiating or maintaining a healthy well-balanced diet that is low in saturated fats, contains moderate levels of lean protein, and is higher in low glycemic fruits and vegetables will reduce the risk of developing these health issues, and when rigorously adhered to, can significantly reduce the impact of the disorder itself. For example, eating a diet that is rich in whole grains, fruits, vegetables and low-fat dairy products that also seriously restricts the use of saturated fats and cholesterol, has been show to reduce blood pressure by up to 14 mm Hg – even more than exercise alone. This eating plan is known as the Dietary Approaches to Stop Hypertension (DASH) diet.

I do not advocate the use of grains in a diet, and prefer individuals follow the Mediterranean or Paleo diet guidelines. These are more consistent and in line the beliefs and assertions of Dr. William Davis, the author of Wheat Belly. He states: "Grains and sugars CAUSE type 2 diabetes. Wheat is the worst of all grains and therefore wheat causes diabetes.: According to Dr. Davis, there are a number of ways that this happens:

1) The complex carbohydrate in wheat, gives it an unusual susceptibility to digestion by the salivary and stomach enzyme, amylase, and raises blood sugar to sky-high levels. Dr. Davis uses the example of two slices of whole wheat bread raising blood sugar higher than 6 teaspoons of table sugar;

2) When blood glucose is high, it then damages pancreatic beta cells that produce insulin;

3) Following the consumption of highly-digestible wheat-based carbohydrates, triglyceride-rich liver fat-based proteins enter the

bloodstream which damages the pancreatic beta cells that produce insulin;

4) Repetitive high blood sugars, such as that developing after a diet rich in "healthy whole grains," via an uncertain cascade of events, including the two detailed above, leads to insulin resistance, that places greater demand on the pancreas to produce more insulin;

5) Insulin resistance triggers the accumulation of visceral fat: muffin top, love handles, or wheat belly;

6) Visceral fat is inflammatory fat that worsens insulin resistance.

In short: wheat consumption = diabetes. Accordingly, no wheat often means no diabetes.

However, neither Dr. Davis nor I are telling you not to eat foods rich in fiber. This is one of the important dietary keys to reducing many health risks, such as high blood pressure, high cholesterol, and has been shown to reduce the risk associated with the development of atherosclerosis. But fiber does not have to come from grains. Many healthful sources of nuts, fruits, seeds, and vegetables are fiber rich, and will not carry the same risks associated with high fiber from whole grains.

Of course, with high blood pressure, there is the need to reduce sodium levels in your diet. Research tells us that even a small reduction in the sodium in your diet can reduce blood pressure by 2 to 8 mm Hg. Limiting salt intake however, does not predicate an automatic loss of flavor in your foods. When cooking, the addition of varied spices and seasonings can open up new horizons and create new tastes that you might never have experienced before.

When I work with clients and discuss dietary changes that appear on the surface to limit their traditional food choices, they initially freak out thinking there is nothing they can eat anymore. The issue I always tell them is this: When we grow up in our homes as children, our mother cooked similar meals or meal patterns on a regular basis, so we we knew only the foods we were exposed to in our home. Then we became adults, perhaps went away to college or when we were first on our own, and we started to venture out a bit from the foods we knew from our youth. Perhaps you tried sushi for the first time, or tofu; perhaps an heirloom tomato – and realized there were more foods available that were really enjoyable. As a result, your frame of reference for what is available to eat increased a little bit. The reality, however, is that there are literally hundreds and hundreds of delicious foods available that you may never have been exposed to that are delicious and healthy. Therefore, while you may have to do without a specific food source or ingredient for your health, particularly if it is associated with preventing the onset or mitigating those risks associated with the development of dementia, your net available food list will actually be significantly larger than you ever imagined before any limitations were placed upon you. It's all a matter of exposure and a willingness to learn. I promise, as my upcoming book *Paleo Basics* discusses, you never have to compromise on taste, texture, or variety just because something is removed from your diet. I assure you, and I invite you to learn as well, *Paleo Basics* will easily demonstrate there need never be a boring moment related to diet or food!

Reduce stress

Stress management is a hugely problematic area for many people. Even for those who devote their lives to and believe in the power of prayer and faith, for many stress is still something that affects us. Additionally, here's a little known fact that you may not be aware of:

any stress, whether positive stress such as the excitement associate with getting engaged or landing a new job, or negative stress such as a divorce or being terminated from a job – they are all interpreted the same way physiologically, and will take a negative toll on your body. What happens is this: Chronic stress exposes your body to unhealthy, persistently elevated levels of stress hormones, such as adrenaline and cortisol which changes the way blood clots, and increases the risk of heart attack. Additionally, and most important to our discussions on cardiovascular risks related to atherosclerosis and other issues, scientists from Massachusetts General Hospital and Harvard Medical School investigating the link between stress and heart attacks reported that stress causes our bodies to make a surplus of disease-fighting white blood cells. The problem is that the white blood cells in this case, can increase inflammation in the arteries of people with a condition called atherosclerosis, where the artery walls are thickened by a build-up of plaque.

There are a number of effective stress management strategies, ranging from simple walking and or exercise, to engaging in hobbies such as painting. Some people enjoy mechanical work, and men might purchase an old car in need of significant repairs that they tinker with every spare moment. For some its home repairs. Whatever you chose to engage in, know this: effective stress management training and use alone has been demonstrated as effective in reducing high blood pressure by stress an average of 2.3 mm Hg, and transcendental meditation or prayer have been reported to reduce blood pressure by more than 5 mm Hg without employing any other stress reduction or blood pressure lowering methods.

Final comments on natural treatments

One of the big challenges I have as a doctor of naturopathy is dispelling the myth that just because something is natural or organically sourced, that it is healthy and good for you. An example I love to use, because it is one of those few absolutes in life goes like this: I often take clients on shopping trips to health food stores to teach them how to read food labels and chose items specific to meet their health needs, and of course what to look for in foods they should not consume. Inevitably, when we get to the isle that has organic chocolate bars they ALL, without exception, believe they can still have one. "But it says it's all natural, look, it's even made with organic sugar— "I think you get my point. NOT EVERYTHING NATURAL WILL BE HEALTHY FOR YOU!

Similarly, taking the point one step farther, just like pharmaceuticals, some items may be good for you but not for someone else; or they may be good for another person, but not for you.

What do I mean? What am I trying to explain?

In the last chapter it may have seemed to you like I was detailing all the pharmaceuticals associated with a specific risk factor related to the development of dementia. Believe it or not, I wasn't, but it seemed like there were hundreds and hundreds, I know. Well, as you've seen, the same is true for natural health products. And in fact, many natural products are healthful as remedies for more than one area of concern, such as magnesium or 5-HTP.

Think about the last health food store you were in. Like most, they had entire isles or shelves devoted to weight loss products, sections for heart or cardiovascular health (where you'd find items for blood pressure and atherosclerosis), sections for diabetes and sugar control, sections for smoking cessation, and so forth. And that's in addition to the standard alphabetical herbal section, and separate section where homeopathic remedies are provided. In other words, there are hundreds upon hundreds of different natural and organic products available to mitigate the risks we're discussing in this book associated with the onset of dementia.

However, as with pharmaceuticals, (and this gets back to my comments above about natural and organically sourced chocolate bars), just because an item is on the shelf of a health foods store, does not mean it is the specific complex or single ingredient specifically needed for you! How do you know if it is or not? Much like you go to your traditional doctor for a prescription, you go to a qualified naturopathic doctor who knows your situation and has been properly trained to discern the right product or set of products specifically for you. Not for your mother, not for your aunt, not for your best friend, not for your neighbor, but for your unique health history and physiology.

And I do have to add a comment here. When most people go into a health food store and look on the shelves with that look of "what is the best product" on their face, or the "I have no idea what I'm looking at" look, staff are schooled only by their store manager in coming to your rescue and offering help. ***PLEASE,*** I implore you, do not accept help from these individuals as to what you should or should not take. The majority have absolutely no schooling in anything other than what product representatives might have told one manager who might have told another staff member, or they overheard someone mentioning a specific product that fit the needs of someone else. In fact, a major chain of health food stores when I first started practicing as a naturopath, hired a woman (who became a client of mine) who's career had been in retail furniture sales. With no other training in healthcare or natural health, she was hired as their supplement manager! So, case in point. For all you know that person's last job was selling shoes and now they're expected to recommend health supplements for someone. This is a situation that truly frightens me.

That individual does not know your entire health history. That individual does not know what else you are taking, whether supplement or prescription. That individual does not know all the warnings and interactions of diet, supplements, and prescriptions that may or may not be affected by what they recommend. That individual is being irresponsible and putting you and anyone else they seek to help in danger. And more than anything else, that individual does not know nor would they likely understand the 20 pages of contraindications and warnings in the natural medicine guidebook used by myself and many other naturopaths and/or herbalists associated with something as simple as garlic, which is one of the recommended natural remedies that you'll see repeated in this section related to heart health and more!

And this leads me into my last area of caution for this chapter. Just because I am providing a set of remedies that may help lower blood pressure, may help with weight loss, may help with smoking and alcohol cessation, may help with atherosclerosis, and so forth – that does not mean you can go to your nearest health food store either and start taking some of these. Well – I suppose you could; but to take a responsible approach, I implore you to seek your care and recommendations from a qualified natural health professional. At the end of this book my office contact information is provided. I am always happy to consult with anyone to assure they're receiving the best recommendations possible on natural approaches that can help mitigate any risk associated with dementia, or work with any other issue.

Chapter Seven: Putting it all together

Traditionally, the writing, speaking, and client consulting I've done regarding dementia and Alzheimer's disease has been filled with sadness, and to be honest, anguish, focusing on the needs of newly diagnosed patients and knowing the fears they are going through, and questions they have. However, this book has provided a different opportunity for me. Rather than anguish and pain, I sought to provide hope; and not only hope for those struggling with dementia, but proactive hope in educating others on how to prevent becoming a frighteningly growing statistic as both the rates of dementia and Alzheimer's disease are dramatically increasing, as is the death rate specifically from dementia and Alzheimer's disease.

As a naturopath, and medical researcher and scientist, I believe in proactive healthcare. I am also keenly aware of major chronic illnesses plaguing our society, as those are primarily what I deal with in my private practice. When putting the puzzle pieces together, it was easy to see that, in addition to being major risk factors for the onset of dementia, many of these chronic illnesses were starting to affect children in record numbers never seen before.

By analyzing these issues, and realizing that the 300% anticipated growth rate for Alzheimer's disease alone over the next 35 years, not counting the other dementias, is essentially a generation, we know that children and young adults are being predisposed to the onset in their senior years, by their own chronic illnesses affecting them now.

So – what do we have?

We already have a generational curse related to Alzheimer's disease - if an individual has a parent diagnosed with Alzheimer's, they are already 25% more likely than an individual who's parent does not have this disorder to become victimized in their own later years.
We already know that for those carrying the APEO-e4 gene, they are genetically predisposed to a 20 – 25% greater risk factor of developing Alzheimer's than their peers who do not possess the gene, and those with specific protein structures, amyloid precursor protein (APP), presenilin-1 (PS-1), and presenilin-2 (PS-2) carry a 5% increased risk. And these figures are in addition to the 25% greater risk carried when a parent has been diagnosed with Alzheimer's disease or one of the other dementias.

But what about all the other risk factors predisposing one to the onset of dementia or specifically Alzheimer's disease? As you've' seen in this book, there are several core risk factors, such as atherosclerosis, high blood pressure, high cholesterol, obesity, smoking, emotional disorders, and heavy metal toxicity. Although many of these are viewed differently by the traditional medical community from those practicing natural healthcare, the issues exist nonetheless, and should be proactively addressed. If one proactively addresses a risk, and can mitigate that risk, the likelihood of a problem arising is significantly lower.

If you can mitigate the risks associated with the development of any of the dementias, including Alzheimer's disease, then you no longer need worry about becoming a statistic.

And, if you address this issue as a young adult, and with your children or grandchildren, you can easily break that generational 25% risk factor that exists, which I strongly believe will only increase as the years progress as a natural statistical outgrowth of children growing into chronically ill adults who grow into chronically ill seniors who then develop dementia or Alzheimer's disease. As the anticipated growth factor for diagnosed cases is projected to increase by 300% over the next 35 years, I believe the corresponding level of 25% of cases where parents diagnosed with one of the dementias have offspring later diagnosed with the same condition will also increase dramatically – unless people take a proactive preventative position.

As I've said throughout this book, even as a naturopath, I strongly believe there is a proper time for taking prescription medicine. I've detailed the reasons in Chapter Four, and I've also provided lists of various pharmaceuticals used to treat the chronic conditions that are considered risk factors associated with the onset of dementia. Chapter Five followed the same process providing natural treatments for the same, and several other risk factors. Potential side effects and areas of caution and concern were also provided for each, whether pharmaceutical or natural treatment.

The difference, however, is if one is predisposed to any of the risk factors, barring any contraindications, many natural preventative treatments can also be employed proactively to prevent atherosclerosis, or diabetes, or high cholesterol, for example. And, certainly addressing these issues with children and young adults, to create healthy habits including a healthy diet and lifestyle incorporating regular exercise are critical to breaking the growing generational curse known as dementia.

As a final note, for those interested in learning more about any of the topics presented in this book, I would be very happy to discuss these in greater length. The same is true for those already diagnosed, or with family members already diagnosed with dementia or Alzheimer's disease who are in the early stages, and wish to learn more about natural treatment options. In fact, in addition to the book *Paleo Basics*, the upcoming book *Treating Dementia, Naturally* will specifically address treating dementia naturally. Believe it or not, it can be done, and successfully!

About the Author

Dr. West-Stellick is a much sought after naturopath with clients literally throughout the world. When not working directly with clients, Dr. West is a well respected writer, lecturer, and seminar leader.

After spending upwards of 30 years in corporate America in a variety of management positions, Dr. West-Stellick's passion for medicine overcame her business success and she received a doctorate of natural healthcare, establishing and maintaining a very successful practice for 17 years, subsequently spending another 10 years as a medical ghostwriter and researcher. Dr. West is the author of over 25 books on a wide variety of topics, for both the secular and Christian market, including: *Ten Essential and Simple Steps to Managing Your Doctor: Empowering you, the Patient; Ten Essential and Simple Steps to Becoming Your Own Case Manager: A Guide for Handling Multiple Medical Issues; Authentic, Inspired, Inerrant, and True; In Sickness and in Health; God, Marriage, and Illness; The God Prescription; Fear of Forgetting Jesus; My Life, My Memories; Preventing Dementia Naturally: Assuring the healthy child, adult, and senior throughout the generations; Treating Dementia, Naturally; Paleo Basics; Paleo-licious Pasta; The Paleo Pup;* and *The Kegel Myth.*

Other Lariat Publishing Books by Dr. Danielle West-Stellick

Ten Essential and Simple Steps to Managing Your Doctor: Empowering you, the Patient
Ten Essential and Simple Steps to Managing your Doctor: Empowering You, the Patient provides a wealth of information in easy to follow segments that will transition you from being the passive patient to the empowered patient, from waiting and being at the mercy of the medical system to the patient who takes responsibility for their healthcare and their life as they seek to form a partnership with their physician. The Ten Essential and Simple Steps to Managing Your Doctor: Empowering You, the Patient is written in an easy to follow workbook format, including pages you can scan or photocopy and use as is or adapt for your own use. For other situations discussed, such as reaching your physician when you have questions or even emergency situations and need to speak with him, sample scenarios are written out in script fashion, providing the framework for your own adaptation to your specific situations as needed. ISBN: 978-1887219211

Ten Essential and Simple Steps to Becoming Your Own Case Manager: A Guide for Handling Multiple Medical Issues
Keeping track of one health issue is sometimes enough to make a person crazy! Juggling multiple health challenges can be impossible! The ten very simple steps in this book help you become your own case manager, help you organize and keep track each illness and the doctors involved. The steps in this book also helps you maintain a position of authority and strength while assuring all doctors involved in each piece of the puzzle that is uniquely you, are communicating effectively with a complete and comprehensive flow of information among and between all parties providing any level of care for you. This is in workbook format, inclusive of forms and pages you may wish to scan or photocopy and use. ISBN: 978-1887219228

Authentic, Inspired, Inerrant, and True
From the beginning, Satan has attempted to make us question God's Word to us. Part of Satan's plan is to cause us to doubt that the Bible is God's authentic, inspired, inerrant and true message to us all. It's easier to look at the Bible as a storybook or piece of literature rather than know God's Word is the truth. Thus, many people think of the Bible as a storybook of a book of historical literature -

therefore, whether it is true or not is immaterial. Many people say they believe in parts of the Bible, but not others. We know that the Bible is authentic, inspired, inerrant and true Word of God: if part is true, all is true. If all of God's word is true, we must face the truth about our own moral character. Thus, through independent research and with the goal of Scripture proving Scripture rather than relying on what man says about God's Word, this book gradually came together exploring such topics as: what God says, statistical proof, historical and archeological evidence, and prophecy. And finally, we look at how the various versions of the Bible came about and a candid discussion is provided on how accurate or inaccurate they today's Bibles are. Let Dr. West-Stellick lead you on an exciting journal that lays the foundation, and then covers 3,500 years of writing, translations, discoveries and more. *Authentic, Inspired, Inerrant and True* will bring you to the fact-based conclusion: The Bible IS God's Word to us. ISBN: 978-1887219105

In Sickness and in Health
In Sickness and in Health represents raw emotion. Inside you will find friends who have experienced what happens when chronic illness becomes the uninvited third member in your marital relationship. Inside, patients share their stories of pain and regret; partners and spouses share their frustrations, and fears. Both share the experiences of unplanned changes to their relationship. All share stories that are all too common when people gloss over the "In Sickness and in Health" part of their wedding vows, and reality sets in when someone is diagnosed with a life-altering chronic illness. This book provides a key message to all patients and partners: you are not alone. Others have walked (or been wheeled) in your shoes. *In Sickness and in Health* provides the unique ability to learn what your partner is likely to be thinking and why he or she is behaving in a specific way that you may not know about. This book does not promise to transform your relationship, but it does promise to leave you with the knowledge that you are not alone in your journey. ISBN: 978-1887219204

God, Marriage, and Illness
It is a sobering truth. The divorce rate for physically healthy couples is between 40-50 %, the divorce rate for those plagued by chronic illness is in excess of 75 percent. When illness strikes, suddenly most people wonder what happened to that wonderful, caring, sensitive person they fell in love with. They wonder why they feel alone, and why they hurt even though they are still married or in a significant relationship. They wonder why their Godly marriage is falling apart. Part of the problem is focus. When there is a lack of reliance on God once illness presents in a marriage, the Illness, Marriage, and God paradigm needs to be transformed into one that places God first, followed by your marriage, and then,

and only then, the focus on illness should enter into the triad. With the rate of chronic illnesses increasing at an alarming rate, readers must take action and INVEST to protect or repair their marriage in only the way that dependence and a focus on God can provide! What *God, Marriage, and Illness* offers is an interactive workbook designed to enable the reader a way to regain the proper perspective and focus on God first in their life. ISBN: 978-188721920242

The God Prescription
Despite professional medical evidence that stresses prayer and attention to the spiritual life of a chronically ill patient dramatically serves to improve their quality of life, upwards of 72% of all healthcare professionals never broach the subject with their patients, opting to focus instead on the medical model of patient care. Sadly, the traditional medical model draws the patient's attention away from the spiritual Godly realm and focuses it on the patient themselves. The real focus need to remain on Him, not the self. *The God Prescription* puts the focus back on God. *The God Prescription* can help you to: 1. Enhance your quality of life; 2. Reduce chronic pain and inflammation; 3. Transform limitations into opportunities that glorify God; and 4. Draw you closer to God. Writing from personal experience as a doctor and as a patient, Dr. West brings you: *The God Prescription.* ISBN: 978-1887219020

Fear of Forgetting Jesus
Building the The Christian edition of *Fear of Forgetting*, which delves into the heart and soul of a person diagnosed with Alzheimer's disease or one of the dementias as virtually every area of their life is examined. Following a detailed presentation of the physiology involved in the disease progression, with the help of scripture, areas of the individual's life are examined along with probing questions requiring the patient to document their feelings and experiences, along with their questions regarding risks, how they feel about memory loss and issues related to making new memories, including a major section delving into who the patient thinks Jesus is, their relationship with Jesus, familial history and experiences, favorite prayers, favorite scriptures, and more. A detailed exploration of generational curses and sin are also incorporated, as is a strong focus on prayer and the development of a prayer life that can transcend their journey. Like *Fear of Forgetting, Fear of Forgetting Jesus* guides the reader past their diagnosis and provides important information in an easy to understand way that educates the patient about what is really happening to their brain, what the journey will be like, and what they can do about their diagnosis to embrace their journey. *Fear of Forgetting Jesus* is also purposely designed to enable easy reading for the older individual already in the early stages of the disease; in workbook format, it guides the patient through an introspective

process of examining and documenting their fears, thoughts, and emotions about the diagnosis, the journey they will take, and *how they believe it will be best to reach them* as the disease progresses based on their unique life events, likes, and dislike, and should become a living journal for family and friends to use as a non-threatening springboard for discussion and care. And like *Fear of Forgetting, Fear of Forgetting Jesus* also includes the free bonus: *My Life, My Memories*, a special memory prompting diary all about who you are! ISBN: 978-1887219273

My Life, My Memories
My Life, My Memories is a journal for completion by the dementia patient This journal will prompt you to write out answers to questions about your life, and your memories. The goal is to achieve a comprehensive book of your life, who you are, and what you are most likely to remember most as Alzheimer's disease or one of the other dementias progress. This journal will tie the patient's current life and past (stored memories) together. It will also help others to work with the patient in the later stages of the disease when, based on the patient's responses to the prompts in this book, for example, when you state likes and dislikes not only from the present but from the past. Topics covered include general information (such as your name), work history, education, romance, childhood and teen years, religion, food, and a section called "last but not least" where the patient can enter anything else that may have been overlooked but is considered by the patient to be important!
ISBN: 978-1887219327

Paleo Basics: A delicious guide to what Paleo is all about, and how to become a Paleo Pro in no time!
Paleo Basics is designed to provide a wealth of information on the why's and how to's of starting on the Paleo Diet, filling in many of the gaps left in other books. For example, in Part One, *Paleo Basics* starts out explaining what the Paleo Diet is, and why a person should follow it, then goes on to discuss the finer points one needs to know in order to really make the Paleo Diet a lifestyle change. For example, setting up the Paleo kitchen, what is a Paleo grocery list like and how to construct one, how to grocery shop, and so forth. Then we talk about how to maintain a social life and remain on the Paleo Diet. Part Two picks up with super easy, delicious, and versatile recipes ranging from appetizers and breakfast dishes to sauces, snacks, and baked goods. This book is a must have to answer all the most common questions about going Paleo, and more than that, guides you through easy Paleo recipes that will ensure you can become a Paleo Pro in no time at all!
ISBN: 978-1887219471

Paleo-licious Pasta! The definitive Paleo Pasta cookbook
Paleo-licious Pasta can give back the joy of pasta to those believed that following the Paleo diet completely removed that from the realm of pasta-bility! Part One details 10 different pasta recipes, ranging from the how-to's of making basic noodles to going beyond the basics with recipes for beet, tomato, spinach, and butternut squash pastas. Part Two provides over 50 exciting Paleo pasta recipes ranging from Paleo Mac N'Cheese to Turkey Tetrazzini. There's even a section on dessert pasta, including Paleo chocolate pasta in custard sauce, sweet Paleo noodle pudding, and Paleo strawberry pasta in lemon custard.
ISBN: 978-1887219488

The Paleo Pup
More and more and more veterinarians and veterinary bloggers are advocating raw and grain-free diets for their dog. As a result, healthful dog food and dog treat manufacturers are supplying raw and grain-free products. With this in mind, Part One of The Paleo Pup examines the health issues surrounding raw and grain-free feeding, and Part Two provides a wide raw and grain-free recipes to delight your pet!
ISBN: 978-1887219495

The Kegel Myth
Pelvic floor problems, characterized by poor bladder control and often a prolapsed bladder or uterus is a common problem experienced by millions of women throughout the world, affecting every one out of three to four women, yet it is a topic considered taboo for polite society and rarely discussed. Additionally, pelvic floor problems can become draining on women and affect our daily lives than most are willing to admit. Perhaps you've even joked about it, and maybe have had to cross your legs when you laugh, cough or sneeze. For some, they're no longer able to play with their children or grandchildren jumping on trampolines or playing jump-rope because they know what will happen. Women everywhere seem to rush to the restroom but pretend it's normal. However, the problem extends past urinary incontinence into our intimate lives. And the good news is that all of these issues can be reversed within two weeks or even prevented with proper exercise, emphasis on "proper." And by proper, we don't mean the *just clench* exercise model of the Kegel Exercise today. That only includes one part of Dr. Kegel's program developed over 70 years ago that achieved 90% success! Just "doing your Kegel's" as currently recommended is not enough! It isn't the "proper exercise!" In fact, the exercise that you see today called a Kegel exercise bears very little resemblance to the actual exercise Dr. Kegel treated his patients with. ISBN: 978-1887219501

Consultations provided worldwide via Skype. Please leave a message on my Facebook page link below

Be sure to LIKE us on Facebook:

https://www.facebook.com/Dr-Danielle-West-ND-Naturopathic-Healthcare-201497746608979/

All publications are available on Amazon throughout the world!

Made in the USA
Monee, IL
08 November 2026

67377617R00070